Healing and Revitalizing
Your Vital Organs

Other Books by the Author

Helping Your Health With Enzymes

Magic Minerals: Key to Better Health

The Natural Way to Health Through Controlled Fasting

Carlson Wade's Gourmet Health Foods Cookbook

Natural and Folk Remedies

The Natural Laws of Healthful Living

Health Tonics, Elixirs and Potions for the Look and Feel of Youth

Natural Hormones: The Secret of Youthful Health

Health Secrets From the Orient

Magic Enzymes: Key to Youth and Health

The Miracle of Organic Vitamins for Better Health

Miracle Protein: Secret of Natural Cell-Tissue Rejuvenation

All-Natural Pain Relievers

How to Achieve Fast, Permanent Weight Loss With the New Enzyme-Catalyst Diet

Brand Name Handbook of Protein, Calories and Carbohydrates

Slimfasting—The Quick "Pounds Off" Way to Youthful Slimness

Healing and Revitalizing Your Vital Organs

Carlson Wade

Foreword by William S. Keezer, M.D.

Parker Publishing Company, Inc.

West Nyack, New York

© 1978, *by*

PARKER PUBLISHING COMPANY, INC.

West Nyack, N.Y.

Library of Congress Cataloging in Publication Data

Wade, Carlson
    Healing and revitalizing your vital organs.

    Includes index.
    1. Naturopathy. 2. Rejuvenation. 3. Organs
(Anatomy) I. Title.
RZ440.W26   615'.535   78-2787
ISBN 0-13-384354-8

Printed in the United States of America

Dedicated to Your Rejuvenated Face and Body

Foreword by a Doctor of Medicine

Every practicing physician would like to spend more time with each patient, to discuss in detail what is wrong, offer suggestions that will help soothe the health problem, keep the problem from becoming worse, and eliminate the need for constant return visits.

But time forces most physicians to be brief and impersonal. An office or hospital visit is often a hurried experience, sometimes at the expense of the patient's health.

Because doctors lack the time to talk in great detail with each patient, it is a welcome relief to have available Carlson Wade's *Healing and Revitalizing Your Vital Organs.* Here, in one volume, you will find an answer to almost every question you have wanted to ask about your health. Carlson Wade has wisely directed attention to the most pressing health problem of our times—the body organs.

Now, together in one volume for the first time, all body organs are discussed in complete detail, with full home programs and case histories.

This book describes hundreds of natural healing remedies that many people need but cannot ask about in a doctor's office. Having Carlson Wade's *Healing and Revitalizing Your Vital Organs* is just like having a family doctor in your own home for immediate consultation.

In this book, you are told about highly important, but little-known "distress signals." You are given step-by-step programs to create "at home" healers for hundreds of different health problems for all of your body organs.

Carlson Wade has written the most helpful book on natural healing that is currently available. A treasure of information is now available at your fingertips. In your own home, you can enjoy speedy revitalization using fruits, vegetables, juices, grains, water therapy, heat therapy, inhalation therapy, self-massage, and finger-pressure methods.

Each chapter of *Healing and Revitalizing Your Vital Organs* is worth ten visits to the doctor because of the valuable help and advice it offers.

Owning Carlson Wade's book enables you to turn to it first for help and speedy healing of hundreds of common and uncommon ailments related to body organ distress. Here is where you'll look for advice and programs to help relieve allergies, soothe your digestive organs, improve your hearing, "wash your kidneys," protect yourself from gallstones, ease "change of life" symptoms, control a restless pancreas, regulate sugar metabolism, rejuvenate your heart, and wash away cholesterol so that your arteries feel young again.

These body organ healers are described in programs that offer you quick and speedy relief. These programs are for ailments that your family doctor probably has no time to discuss with you. Or else the cost involved would be more painful than the ailment!

Keeping you out of your doctor's office is the greatest benefit of Carlson Wade's book.

Carlson Wade writes in clear, everyday language that you probably wish could be used by the busy physician in his office. This book is like having the 30 minutes you would like to spend with your doctor in a leisurely chat about your health problems.

SPECIAL BONUS: An Organ-Healer Locater Index. Just look up the organ in question in the special index. You can instantly see the healing program and where to find it in the book. The help you want is available at your fingertips.

This book gives you a "complete health blueprint" for a more youthful and energetic life.

William S. Keezer, M.D.

What This Book Will Do for You

This book was written to help keep you out of a doctor's office!

In recent times, doctors are seeing more and more people with sorrowful complaints about their various body organs. Complaints range from indigestion and constipation to poor eyesight, weak hearing, and kidney, liver, and colon disorders. The list is endless. The pain and discomfort keeps on without relief, day and night, around the clock.

These troubled folks are routinely given chemical treatments that open up a Pandora's box of side effects (often more painful than the ailment). This leads to recurring pains, addiction to medicines, and skyrocketing medical bills.

Do you—or a relative or friend—feel you are "at the end of your rope" with this unhealthy (and unhealing) cycle? Then this book is your opportunity to discover how you, in the privacy of your own home, can use natural remedies and drug-free programs to create speedy, effective and long-lasting healing of any or all of your body organs.

That is the purpose and benefit of this book—to keep you OUT of your doctor's office. To keep you AWAY from harmful drugs and medicines. To help you AVOID endless medical bills.

For the first time, there is a book that offers you a treasury of effective, non-surgical, drug-free, natural healing advice for *all of your body organs.* From head to toe, you can adjust and stimulate these "youth motors" so that they can reward you with vitality and bubbling good health.

Here are some of the hundreds of nagging health problems discussed, together with healing and revitalizing home remedies:

Mental Sluggishness	Constipation
Physical Weakness	Diarrhea
Brain Fatigue	Diverticulosis
Nervous Disorders	Stomach Cramps
Premature Aging	Hemorrhoids
Prostate Disorders	Colds
"Shakes"	Nasal Congestion
Aging Skin	Emphysema

Blemishes	Asthma
Heart Complaints	Bronchitis
Arteriosclerosis	Visual Disorders
Hearing Problems	Pancreas Weakness
Liver Ailments	Colon Misbehavior
Kidney Disorders	Inactive Thyroid
Gallstones	"Change of Life"
Indigestion	Ulcers
Fatigue	Dizziness

Would you like a family doctor who:

- Will discuss problems and help you without an appointment?
- Is available for house calls upon a moment's notice at any hour of the day or night?
- Gives you all the time you need to explain (in words you understand) how to heal ailments affecting men, women, youngsters, and elderly people?
- Helps to heal your ailments without drugs or surgery?
- Does not send you an exorbitant bill?

Difficult to believe? Well, it's true. This personal help is now available whenever you need it without your having to leave your home. *Healing and Revitalizing Your Vital Organs* is just that all-purpose family medical guide.

This book shows you how to correct the CAUSE of organ ailments and thereby help relieve symptoms. Your body and mind are rewarded with total health and youthful vitality.

Here are just a few examples of some nagging organ ailments that can be pampered, soothed, and healed with the helpful programs presented in this book:

Aging Skin. Your largest body organ can be refreshed and revitalized with steam treatments, homemade "youth creams," wrinkle erasers, and cell-feeding foods.

Heart Distress. Strengthen and revitalize this "master organ" with special food programs, easy-to-do exercises to improve its rhythm, and circulation-boosting remedies to add years to its life.

Irregularity. Discover how everyday foods can banish constipation within a day or two. Say goodbye to habit-forming laxatives that weaken your organs of elimination. Say hello to tasty foods that strengthen your colon so that you can enjoy daily regularity.

Vision Weakness. Try easy eye exercises and strengthen your sight organs so that you will not have to squint so often. Try a finger-pressure eye massage. Eat tasty foods that nourish your organs of vision.

Gallbladder Rebellion. Tame this organ with natural programs to improve its fat-dispersion ability. Use homemade remedies to protect against inflammation, gallstones, and gallbladder pain. Try the easy gallbladder "cleansing" program that rejuvenates this organ and the entire body.

Painful Stomach Ulcers. Free your stomach from wrenching pains and agonizing "knots" with a collection of easy-to-follow, natural home remedies. Many are so amazingly effective that you will feel relief in just minutes. Ulcer pains are often erased for good with these easy, fast, effective, natural healers.

Fatigue and Weakness. Revitalize the organs that can supercharge your body with youthful energy. Feel alert, invigorated, and revitalized when you stimulate these organs with natural remedies. Many of them will make you feel more alert almost immediately after use.

This book will help children, young adults, middle-aged people, and elderly people—anyone who wants youthful vitality and a longer and healthier life. This book is unique because it is devoted exclusively to your internal and external organs, those little-known, but vital "power stations" of your body. These organs are like intricately patterned printed circuits within your human machine. Each one is part of a chain and works in harmony with other organs to reward you with total health.

But note this carefully: The malfunctioning of just one organ can break down the entire chain. Just one weak link can cause the collapse of your entire body. That is why this book was written, to show you how to revitalize your body links, your body organs, which are the very foundation of your health. This book shows you how to alert your body organs so that they can work in harmony. Your human machine will then throb with vitality and youthful health.

Before you try anything drastic, before you helplessly agree to surgery, before you accept drugs that can cause painful side effects, you owe it to yourself to give your body a chance with any of the hundreds of natural healers included in this book. This book presents a variety of safe alternatives that offer hope for total body health through organ revitalization.

Above all, this book was written with *your* needs in mind. Keep it available for immediate use. The help offered by this book may be a welcome turning point in the health of many who use it. One such revitalized person can be you!

Carlson Wade

Table of Contents

Healing and Revitalizing
Your Vital Organs

How to Refresh and Revitalize Your Body with Natural Youth Serum

1

From head to toe, your body can be refreshed and revitalized so that you radiate the joys of looking and feeling youthful and healthy. This dynamic internal supercharging of vigor and vitality is altered through the action of a set of six closely connected "master time-pieces" known as glands. When you alter the natural life forces within your body, these six master timepieces wind up and then release an around-the-clock supply of "youth serums" known as hormones. These all-natural youth serums bathe, nourish, and rejuvenate almost all parts of your body, both emotionally and physically. When these six master timepieces are wound up, they have the power to send forth these youth serums, which spring to your defense, protecting you against illness and creating a natural life force that will help you enjoy youthful health of body and mind.

YOUR GLANDS: "MASTER TIMEPIECES" OF YOUTHFUL HEALTH

Endocrine (ductless) glands are so named because their youth serums (hormones) do not pass through ducts or tubes but pour directly into the bloodstream, where they participate in almost every emotional and physical function. These master timepieces influence the appearance of your skin, determine your weight, regulate your metabolism, give you energy, protect you against illness, shield you against the aging factor, and fill you with the joy of youthful life.

You have six basic glands in your body. They work in harmony.

To furnish the youth serums known as hormones, these glands are part of a giant internal chain link. Like closely connected master timepieces, each one depends upon the other for smooth functioning and revitalization of the body. If there is a weakness in one of these timepieces, the others start to weaken and falter in their secretion of the youth serums. That is why it is important to keep all six of your master timepieces in good health. Like a natural *computer right in your body,* these master timepieces are interconnected and work in harmony to enrich your life with the endowment of youthful health. As this chapter will describe, you can wind up each and every one of your master timepieces so that your "biological computer" can send forth an around-the-clock supply of youth serums.

YOUR HORMONES: "YOUTH SERUMS" FOR PERPETUAL HEALTH

Your body glands rejuvenate every component of your physical and emotional being by secreting substances known as hormones, or youth serums. The word *hormone* is derived from the Greek word *hormaein,* meaning "to excite." These hormones actually do "excite" the body so that all of your functions are alerted and activated. These youth serums influence your growth and development, tissue and cell repair, fertility, muscular tone, energy, digestion and metabolism, and resistance to and ability to fight ill health. Most important, a steady supply of youth serums can help guard against aging and help you look and feel young!

These youth serums work in harmony. That is, your glands act as part of a giant internal computer. There are communication mechanisms between these glands so that they can work together to continuously nourish your vital organs and reward you with good health. In order for them to do this, you need to keep your glands nourished and healthy so they can secrete adequate amounts of youth serums at the proper, balanced levels.

To tap the dynamic life force within your body and to help revitalize your body and mind, keep your master timepieces nourished so they send forth a refreshing and steady stream of youth serums.

To heal and revitalize all of your body organs, begin with your six basic glands.

MASTER TIMEPIECE #1—PITUITARY GLAND

Location: Pea-sized, the pituitary hangs from a short stalk at the base of the brain.

Youth Serum: The pituitary consists of three lobes, which secrete at least 12 known youth serums or hormones. These three lobes and their youth serums are as follows.

Posterior Lobe. The posterior lobe secretes youth serums that activate smooth muscular function, regulate water balance, stabilize kidney function and guard against problems of diabetes.

Anterior Lobe. Located opposite the posterior lobe, the anterior lobe secretes youth serums that maintain normal height, promote milk production from within the female breast, help store and distribute fat and also guard against weight irregularities.

Intermediate Lobe. Centrally located, the intermediate lobe secretes a youth hormone that determines skin color. It influences skin texture and youthfulness and is also influential in nourishing cells with adequate moisture to protect against unnecessary wrinkling.

As the master timepiece of all the glands, the pituitary gland needs to be healthy and well-nourished to secrete its vital youth serums.

A Pituitary-Feeding Program for Total Revitalization

To nourish, as well as oxygenate, your pituitary gland so it can secrete youth-maintaining serums, a simple feeding program has been devised to give it the necessary working materials. Following is this easy-to-follow program.

Early Morning Brain Breathing Booster: A sluggish pituitary gland, especially in the morning, can spell disaster for the day or even all week. This was the problem faced by Bertha A., an over-60 housewife and part-time office bookkeeper. She felt sluggish and mentally exhausted in the morning and had to gulp down cup after cup of coffee to stay alert. The caffeine in the coffee, though, whipped up her pituitary gland and made her so nervous that she was jittery for most of the day. A friend who was a physiotherapist told her to "kick the coffee habit." To revitalize her sluggish pituitary gland, Bertha A. replaced coffee with the physiotherapist-recommended *Early Morning Brain Breathing Booster.*

Upon awakening, slowly swing your legs onto the floor. While sitting on your bed, head held comfortably high, gently take a deep breath. Then count one. Now exhale as you count two. Repeat this step by taking a deep breath as you count three and then exhale as you count four. Repeat this procedure until you have reached the count of 20.

Benefit: A sluggish pituitary is "choked" for lack of oxygen which has been reduced during sleeping time. During sleep, oxygen is drawn from the brain to the digestive region. This permits the brain to become "sluggish" to allow sleep. But, upon awakening, the oxygen-starved brain requires a fresh flow of "breath" to nourish its pituitary lobes so they can secrete their youth serums. When you follow this easy *Early Morning Brain Breathing Booster,* a new supply of oxygen is sent streaming to the lobes. The oxygen carries stored-up nutrients that nourish the pituitary gland so it can pour forth vitality-producing youth serums and give you an alert and active brain.

Bertha A. followed this simple five-minute program every morning and discovered that it energized her from head to toe with more lasting (more healthful) results than the coffee did. Now she has the vitality of a youngster as she does her housework and her office work.

Protein-Plus Pituitary Tonic. Meet the challenges of stress and tension by fortifying your pituitary with two basic nutrients—protein and Vitamin C. Prepare a tasty *Protein-Plus Pituitary Tonic* by stirring two tablespoons of unflavored gelatin powder into a glass of grapefruit juice. Stir until the gelatin is completely dissolved. Then drink this tonic slowly. Drink a glass whenever you anticipate a particularly stressful situation. You may also drink a glass of this tonic when you find yourself very upset, especially following a stressful occurrence.

Benefit: The Vitamin C of the grapefruit juice is activated by its enzymes, which then take up the protein of the gelatin powder and send it to the pituitary gland. Here, your metabolism uses the transformed protein together with Vitamin C to alert the pituitary to secrete more of its youth serums. The pituitary issues ACTH and STH, two *protective* hormones that act as insulators to shield you from the shock of stress and tension. Without these two youth serums, you could not expect to cope with the stress of everyday living. Drink the *Protein-Plus Pituitary Tonic* before, during and after any stressful situation, and you'll enable the youth serums to create a buffer zone so that you can cheerfully cope with the conditions.

Fruit Fast for Pituitary Power. As an office supervisor, Michael T. became the victim of recurring "brain fatigue." Numbers looked jumbled on his papers. Words came out slurred. His reflexes were slow. Michael T. made costly mistakes that threatened his job. He was unjustly labelled "senile" even though he was only in his early 50's. Michael T. needed something fast to get him out of his "tired brain" syndrome. So he went on a simple one day fruit fast as described in a magazine feature article.

Simple Program: For one day, nourishment consists solely of raw fruits and raw fruit juices. *Breakfast* is a half of grapefruit and a serving of orange, tangerine, pineapple, pear, and banana slices. A citrus fruit juice is the beverage. *Lunch* is a seasonal melon topped with grapes and a serving of berries, raisins, dates, pitted prunes, and figs. A citrus fruit juice is the beverage. *Dinner* is a serving of sun-dried fruits, such as apricots, raisins, and pitted prunes, and seasonal berries, papaya slices, and mango slices. A citrus fruit juice is the beverage.

Benefit: Without interference from heavy fats or protein, the body is able to work efficiently to take the Vitamin C from the raw fruits and juices and transport it via the bloodstream to the brain, where it enters into the construction of collagen, the "cement" that binds cells together. Michael T. discovered that the Vitamin C nourishes the pituitary gland, activating its three-lobed mechanism to secrete a steady supply of the youth serum hormones that amplified his hypothalamus. The hypothalamus is the floor of the front part of the brain between the cerebral hemispheres. It needs Vitamin C to help regulate body functions and make the body active. The *Fruit Fast* that Michael T. followed for just one day gave his pituitary gland the nourishment it needed to rejuvenate his "tired" nervous system.

Soon, Michael T. was able to work with youthful vitality and energy. He follows a *Fruit Fast* at least one day per week for good taste and a natural way to fill his body with the youth serums that transformed him from being "senile" to being "a bundle of energy!"

The pituitary gland, the master timepiece, is the leader of the entire glandular network. For more emotional and physical energy, nourish it with oxygen and healthy foods, and it will secrete all-natural youth serums.

MASTER TIMEPIECE #2–ADRENAL GLANDS

Location: Shaped like Brazil nuts, the adrenal glands are located above each kidney. Each adrenal gland consists of: the *cortex,* or the outer shell, and the *medulla,* or the inner core.

Youth Serum: The medulla sends forth a youth serum known as adrenaline, or *epinephrine,* which alerts the mind and body to meet the responsibilities of daily living. The adrenal glands also secrete *corticosteroid,* a youth serum that builds resistance to disease, gives you strength, cheers you up, and makes life worth living.

An Adrenal-Feeding Program for Total Revitalization

Adrenal glands act like biological computers to give you the answers to the problems that assail you in daily living. To keep these biological computers working at top efficiency, you must keep them "oiled" through good nourishment. Following are basic adrenal-gland-feeding programs.

From "Obsolete" to "Overachiever" in Three Days. Caroline J. found that her nerves were becoming ragged, her energy was short-lived, and her temper was on edge. Supervisors at the large department store where she worked wanted to fire her for being "obsolete," as they cruelly put it. But a kindly salesgirl took Caroline J. aside and told her of a three-day "gland-feeding" program that had transformed her into a bubbly personality. She told Caroline J. how to transform herself in a short time.

Adrenal-Activating Bath-Shower: In the morning, enjoy a soak in comfortably hot water for ten minutes. Then let the water drain out of the tub. Stand up (hold onto support to avoid a fall) in the tub. Turn on the shower to a comfortable warm spray. Let it spray you from head to toe for two minutes. *Slowly* adjust the knobs to cool the water. Enjoy the gland-revitalization of a stinging cold shower for just one minute. All the while rub yourself with a rough washcloth. Turn off the shower. Step out. Dry yourself vigorously.

Benefit: Caroline J. discovered that this *Adrenal-Gland-Activat-*

ing Bath-Shower alerted her senses and gave her unbelievable vitality so that she could face the day with renewed energy. The unique benefit of this bath-shower is that the *contrast* of hot and cold water, together with the vigorous rubbing, alerts the adrenal glands to send forth the youth serum adrenaline to nourish the sympathetic nervous system. This youth serum sends a supply of blood to the body muscles and then boosts the release of glucose (as ready energy) from the liver into the bloodstream. This helps create a feeling of vitality and energy that helps the body and mind work together as a unit of youthful vigor. Caroline J. discovered that this free all-natural program washed away the cobwebs from her mind so that she could face the day with renewed energy.

Feeding Adrenal Glands. Caroline J. then followed the second half of this revitalization program. She gave up all processed and so-called "junk" foods, such as bleached flour products, chemicalized pastries, and cakes. She replaced them with *whole grain* products that were free of additives and without preservatives. Why? Because bleaching grain foods destroys their B vitamins (Vitamin B complex), which are needed by your nervous system. Whole grains are prime sources of B vitamins, which are taken by the body's metabolic system and transported via the bloodstream to the adrenal glands, where they are used to coat the myelin sheath, the covering of the body's network of nerves. The adrenal hormones take the B vitamins and use them to insulate the nervous system so that it is buffered from daily stresses and can meet the challenges of moderate to severe tension.

Three Days Creates a Miracle of Revitalization. In just three days, Caroline J. experienced a total revitalization from head to toe. She felt limitless energy. Her nerve cells could cope with stress. Her senses of sight and hearing were more acute. She could think clearly. Her muscles felt resilient. She felt cheerful, laughed easily, and shrugged good-naturedly when customers argued with her. Caroline J. felt rejuvenated through the revitalization of her adrenal glands. The youth serum adrenalin transformed her from being "obsolete" to being an "overachiever," and she was soon headed for a well-deserved promotion.

The adrenal glands need hot and cold water for activation and the B vitamins from whole grain foods for nerve insulation so that they can secrete an important youth serum that makes life much more beautiful.

MASTER TIMEPIECE #3—THYROID GLAND

Location: The thyroid gland is located in the front of the neck against the wind pipe. It is about two inches long and one-fourth inch wide. It has two parts and resembles a butterfly.

Youth Serum: The thyroid gland releases *thyroxine,* a youth serum that accelerates the release of energy to the tissues from combustion of glucose. When this occurs, respiration and blood circulation are increased to meet the added demand for oxygen. Bodily and mental activities are stimulated. Body temperature is raised to provide warmth to the extremities. Thyroxine is the youth serum the body needs to guard against goiter (enlargement in the thyroid gland) as well as myxedema (middle-aged senility characterized by poor appetite, low energy, aging skin, and dull intellect). With a steady supply of the youth serum thyroxine, the thyroid can help guard against these aging conditions.

A Thyroid-Feeding Program for Total Revitalization

Iodine as "Oil" for the Thyroid Computer. A simple mineral, iodine, is needed as "oil" to lubricate the thyroid computer. When the thyroid receives iodine from food, it stores up as much as it can. This iodine is then released in controlled amounts into the bloodstream. When the bloodstream receives iodine, it uses it to maintain a steady heartbeat, regulate metabolism so there is a steady burning up of foods, guard against goiter, and protect against *myxedema.*

The Seasoning That Becomes a Youth Serum. A tasty and flavorful seasoning known as sea salt, or *kelp,* is a powerhouse of iodine. Available at health food stores, kelp is a powder that is made from dried seaweed. Since the ocean is a source of iodine, any plant or seafood coming from the ocean is also a good source of iodine.

Sprinkle kelp over any foods, raw or cooked, requiring seasoning. Use it as a salt substitute. It is a prime source of the iodine that is needed by your thyroid for use as a vital ingredient in the youth serum thyroxine.

Seafood: Youth Serum from the Oceans. Plan to eat seafood as often as possible. You should schedule it at least three times a week as part of your revitalization plan. Avoid shellfish since these creatures are scavengers that cling to the polluted shores of the rivers and oceans. Instead, select other varieties of ocean fish. They are prime sources of the minerals in the ocean, especially iodine.

Your digestive system takes iodine (along with other nutrients) from the seafood. The iodine is transported via the bloodstream to your thyroid gland, and this master timepiece uses it to transform middle-age into youth. In the form of a youth serum, the iodine is used to create steady energy, stabilize the appetite, moisturize the skin to correct problems of puffiness or dryness, nourish the cells of the brain so thinking is clear and alert, and create feelings of warmth and comfort.

Use sea salt or kelp regularly, eat seafood as often as possible, and boost the action of your thyroid so that it can "keep good time" in your body and mind.

MASTER TIMEPIECE #4—PARATHYROID GLANDS

Location: There are several of these small glands (usually four), which are located behind or embedded in the thyroid gland. Pea-sized, they are situated in the four corners of the thyroid.

Youth Serum: The parathyroid glands release a hormone, a youth serum, that is needed to regulate the concentration of calcium in the blood. This hormone regulates the balance of calcium and phosphorus, which the body uses the strengthen the muscle-nerve network and to strengthen the skeletal system.

A Parathyroid-Feeding Program for Total Revitalization

Strong Bones with Youth Serum. Oscar H. had a strong fear of falling. He was in his early 60's, and he had so-called brittle bones, or osteoporosis. If he fell or bumped himself hard, he ached for days and days, and there was also the risk of a broken bone. To supply his parathyroids with the youth serum needed to build a strong skeleton, his doctor suggested that Oscar H. follow this easy two-step program:

A. *Controlled Sunshine as Often as Possible.* Whenever it was sunny outside, Oscar H. would go for a long, leisurely walk, baring as much of his body to the rays as possible. He carefully kept his head covered, of course. Just an hour of daily sunshine was helpful. *Benefit:* Sunshine activated the oil glands beneath the surface of Oscar H.'s skin to manufacture more Vitamin D, which is important in the construction of the bone system.

B. *Boost Daily Intake of Calcium.* Daily, Oscar H. would drink at least two glasses of skim milk for its high calcium content. He would also nourish himself with other calcium-containing foods, such as

salmon, cabbage, turnips, kale, mustard greens, broccoli, yogurt, and
cheeses. *Benefit:* Oscar H.'s metabolism would take the calcium from
these foods, together with the Vitamin D, manufactured by his skin,
and sift it through the parathyroids to form the parathyroid hormone. This youth serum was then released by the parathyroids to
nourish the bones of the body. The Vitamin D and calcium containing youth serum worked to mineralize the skeletal structure. Soon
Oscar H. felt his entire bone system firming up. His chest was strong.
His hip bones were like those of a flexible youth. His fears of osteoporosis were gone. Now he could work and play with the stamina of a
young man, thanks to the mineralized youth serum that revitalized
and strengthened his skeletal structure.

"Shakes" and "Falling Sickness" Eased with Youth Serum.
Wilma R. was plagued by the "shakes." Her hands and legs trembled
for no reason. Her problems were compounded when she became
increasingly dizzy and developed "falling sickness." Wilma R. wanted
to avoid being confined as an invalid. When a friend who was a nurse
told her that her problems could be traced to a mineral-starved
parathyroid, she decided to follow an easy program outlined by her
friend to correct this condition.

*A Dairy "Fast" with Citrus Juices Lead to the Formation of
Youth Serum.* Wilma R. began by eliminating all artificial, chemicalized, and processed foods from her diet. Then she scheduled a
three-day-per-week Dairy "Fast" for Monday, Wednesday, and
Friday of each week. The gland-feeding fast was simple to follow.
Throughout the day, she drank four glasses of skim milk. At the
same time, she drank citrus fruit juices, such as orange, grapefruit, or
tangerine juice, either singly or in combination.

Benefit: The raw enzymes and Vitamin C in the citrus fruit juices
boost the body's assimilation powers as they take the calcium from
the skim milk and prepare it for the parathyroids. These glands then
take this *energized calcium* and metabolize it into a highly concentrated form of the parathyroid hormone.

The *combination* of dairy enzymes and the Vitamin C in the
citrus juices in a "fast" during which no other foods are taken re-
sulted in a metabolism that could work *free and clear,* without interference, to create the needed parathyroid hormone, or youth serum.

Recovers from "Shakes" and "Falling Sickness." Wilma R. followed this natural program for several weeks. Slowly, her "shakes"
subsided. She no longer experienced vertigo or dizziness; she over-

came her "falling sickness." The tremors and spasms she had felt in her arms and legs now subsided and soon halted all together. Her "agitation" simply disappeared. The youth serum, carrying large amounts of needed calcium, helped cleanse away toxic substances that irritated her brain and nervous system. They neutralized the corrosive reactions of these wastes and then washed them away. Soon, Wilma R. recovered completely. The trembling sensations faded away, and she discovered that life was wonderful, thanks to the youth serum.

MASTER TIMEPIECE #5–PANCREAS

Location: Located behind the stomach, the pancreas is a broad strip of soft glandular tissue. It is broadest on the right where it nestles in the curve of the duodenum (first section of the small intestine). It is wrapped round the portal vein, close to the arteries of the liver and the bile duct.

Youth Serum: The pancreas contains *islets of langerhans,* which release two hormones, insulin and glucagon, that are sent directly into the bloodstream. These hormones regulate the metabolism of sugar and starch. A deficiency of these two youth serums, or hormones, may lead to diabetes.

A Pancreas-Feeding Program for Total Revitalization

To strengthen this gland and nourish it so that is can release sufficient amounts of both insulin and glucagon, it is important to have a balanced diet, but the emphasis here is on the restriction and elimination of refined sugar.

Foods to Avoid: White bread, crackers, noodles, spaghetti, white rice, pizzas, and so on. Sweets, candies, cakes, pies, pastries, doughnuts, and confections. Anything made of or containing white sugar. These foods have been depleted of essential nutrients, and they are high in refined sugar, which places a heavy burden upon the pancreas in its metabolizing responsibility.

Healthy Meat for Pancreas. To nourish the islets of langerhans, buy *stomach sweetbread* from your butcher and eat it several times a week, either baked or broiled. Stomach sweetbread is the pancreas of an animal. *Benefit:* Stomach sweetbread is a prime source of the mineral zinc, which is a nutrient found in insulin. By eating zinc-rich pancreas regularly, you help give your pancreas a powerful supply of zinc, which it needs to secrete natural insulin to metabolize high sugar levels.

Tart, Tangy Fruit for Pancreas. Select a variety of very tart and tangy fruits that nourish the pancreas and do not burden it with the need for much insulin. Such fruits include cranberries, strawberries, tangerines, oranges, lemons, limes, and gooseberries. *Benefit:* Much of the tart fruit's sugar is in the form of fructose, which requires almost no insulin for its metabolism in the body's cells. Some fructose is transformed into glucose during the digestive process, but this is a minimal amount. Since it reduces and eases stress on the pancreas, tart fruit is highly desirable.

Raw Carbohydrates Are Less Burdensome Than Cooked Carbohydrates. Plan to eat raw carbohydrate foods (fruits and vegetables) instead of cooked carbohydrate foods. Raw carbohydrates take a much longer time to reach the bloodstream and are less of a burden on the pancreas. On the other hand, cooked carbohydrates reach the bloodstream as sugar very quickly and force the pancreas to release more insulin in order to metabolize them. This upsets the "time clock" precision of the pancreas, and it is compelled to work at top speed—even overtime. This causes excessive wear and tear on the pancreas and reduces its efficiency. For a healthy pancreas, emphasize the intake of *raw* carbohydrate foods in a balanced diet.

Nourish your pancreas with high-protein foods, eliminate refined sugars and starches from your diet, and drink fresh vegetable juices for good mineral intake. The pancreas will then reward you with the youth serum insulin to metabolize sugars and starches.

MASTER TIMEPIECE #6 (MALE)—PROSTATE

Location: Located at the mouth of the bladder, through which urine is discharged, in men, the prostate has the size and shape of a chestnut.

Youth Serum: The prostate gland releases an alkaline fluid that is a component of male seminal fluid. It determines the fertility of the male. The fluid also nourishes the sperm cells.

A Prostate-Feeding Program for Total Revitalization

Wheat Germ Oil and Vitamin E. These products are prime sources of polyunsaturated fatty acids and Vitamin E, which appear to nourish the cells and tissues of the prostate and thereby boost its ability to manufacture needed sperm cell "youth serums" in the form of seminal fluids. Use wheat germ oil as a dressing on raw vegetable salads. Vitamin E is available in health food stores as a supplement.

Drink Healthy Beverages. Lots of fresh fruit and vegetable juices nourish the prostate with enzymes, vitamins, and minerals. They also help "wash" this gland and keep it free of toxic waste accumulation. Plan to drink at least four glasses of juices daily. They should be at room temperature. *Do not drink iced beverages.* Cold beverages cause a shock to the prostate and upset the timekeeping balance.

How Fred B. Solved Night Bathroom Problems. Troubled by having to get up many times during the night for bathroom trips, Fred B. suffered a loss of health because of his interrupted sleep. He was told by a dietician that he was abusing his prostate with his coffee, tea, and cola drink habit. Fred B. was drinking these beverages throughout the day, even up until bedtime. He made this simple adjustment to solve his having to get up at all hours of the night: He eliminated all coffee, tea and cola drinks. These drinks are high in caffeine, which irritates the prostate and causes forced urination. As a drug, caffeine upsets the delicate balance of this master timepiece, so all forms of caffeine should be eliminated. Replace caffeine drinks with Postum, herbal tea, and fruit or vegetable juices. Fred B. discovered that this simple change in his habits was soothing to his prostate and that he could now enjoy a full night's sleep without disturbance.

European Sitz Bath. European healers recommended the use of a "sitz bath." Sit in a tub of comfortably hot water for about 15 minutes. The water level should reach only to the waistline. Then slowly draw off the hot water and replace it with comfortably cool water. It is said that this contrast in temperature (15 minutes for each) helps soothe the prostate and restore its delicate balance.

Folk Remedy: Folklorists recommend boiling three tablespoons of watermelon seeds in one pint of water, straining them, and then allowing them to cool. Take one teaspoonful of the liquid every hour. The liquid is said to be a prime source of plant proteins and unsaturated fatty acids that appear to nourish the prostate and prompt it to continue releasing its youth serum.

To help revitalize your entire body, keep your prostate healthy. Do this by avoiding alcoholic and other artificially stimulating beverages. Use fresh fruits, vegetables, plant juices, and whole grains. Stay young with a healthy prostate.

MASTER TIMEPIECE #6 (FEMALE)—OVARIES

Location: The ovaries are two small glands, each about the size and shape of an almond, situated in the lower abdomen (pelvic cavity) of women just below the navel. One ovary is about three inches to the right of the center of the body, and the other is about three inches to the left.

Youth Serum: The ovaries release estrogen, the hormone that keeps a woman looking and feeling young. The ovaries also release ova or "egg cells," which determine fertility.

An Ovary-Feeding Program for Total Revitalization

Boost Blood Calcium. Calcium is especially important for soothing the ovaries and nourishing them to guard against malfunctioning. This mineral is found in dairy products (use skim milk products if you are on a fat- or calorie-controlled program) and in plant foods such as apricots, cabbage, mustard greens, and turnips. Plan to drink at least three glasses of milk daily for calcium intake.

Calcium and Vitamin D Help Increase Production of Youth Serum. When calcium is taken together with Vitamin D, there is increased absorption, retention, and utilization of the calcium. In combination, these two nutrients alert and activate the ovaries to release an ample supply of estrogen—its natural youth serum. Calcium appears to be energized and amplified by Vitamin D. *Suggestion:* In a glass of milk, stir two tablespoons of any fish liver oil. Add a bit of honey if desired. Drink the mixture slowly. This mixture is a powerhouse of calcium and Vitamin D, both of which are needed by your ovaries as energizers for them to secrete much-needed youth serum.

Boost Iodine Intake. The ovaries, like the thyroid, contain high concentrations of iodine. This mineral boosts the function of enzymes to keep the ovaries in good working condition. The iodine is in great demand, particularly in older women. To nourish your ovaries with iodine, eat seafoods as often as possible. Also, use sea salt or kelp as a flavoring both in cooking and in the shaker.

With proper health care, the ovaries can be nourished so that they can keep you looking and feeling feminine.

HAPPY GLANDS: GATEWAY TO BODY HEALING

Refresh and revitalize your glands, and you stand at the gateway to total body healing. Happy glands are well-nourished and in efficient condition. They act as master timepieces in your body, producing a steady supply of youth serums. Because the body glands work in harmony, it is beneficial to follow as many of the natural programs I have outlined as possible for total revitalization.

IMPORTANT HIGHLIGHTS

1. To revitalize your organs, begin with your glands. They are your "master timepieces" of youthful health. Nourish them, and they will release a fountain of "youth serums" throughout your body.

2. Bertha A. washed away her exhaustion with an Early Morning Brain Breathing Booster for pituitary alertness. Try a Protein-Plus Pituitary Tonic to boost pituitary release of two important youth serums.

3. Michael T. was transformed from being "senile" to being "a bundle of energy" with a Fruit Fast that boosted pituitary power.

4. Caroline J. went from being "obsolete" to being an "overachiever" by following a three-day adrenal activation program.

5. Iodine helps activate your thyroid for better health and more youth serum.

6. Oscar H. overcame brittle bones by activating his parathyroids through simple nutrition programs.

7. Wilma R. conquered the "shakes" and the "falling sickness" through a special fasting program that caused her parathyroids to secrete important youth serum.

8. Be good to your pancreas and pamper it with tart fruits and special foods that encourage the pancreas to produce its hormones.

9. Fred B. solved glandular "night problems" with a simple program.

10. Women can stay young with healthy ovaries, made possible through the programs outlined in this chapter.

How Home Remedies Can Create Natural "Face Lift" for Forever Young Skin

2

Revitalize your skin—your body's single largest organ—and you will radiate the glow of youth and health. From head to toe, you will enjoy new vitality when the skin is repaired and restored so that it puts roses in your cheeks and gives you the look and feel of youth.

When your skin is properly nourished and cared for, it is smooth, healthy, and the picture of youth. With a variety of home remedies, you can wipe away creases, wrinkles, blemishes, and premature aging signs so that your body's largest organ is a symbol of youthful health.

Skin: Organ of Protection. Your skin serves to protect all that it covers. It protects your body against invasion of bacteria, against injury to the more sensitive tissues within your body, against the rays of the sun, and against the loss of moisture. Your skin serves as an organ of perception for your nervous system. Your skin regulates body temperature. A healthy skin is your first line of defense against the harsh elements that would otherwise cause aging both internally and externally.

The average adult has over 3,000 square inches of surface skin. This skin weighs about six pounds, which is twice as much as the brain or liver. Your skin receives one-third of all of the blood circulating throughout your body. A healthy body begins with healthy skin.

Revitalize Your Two Layers of Skin for Youthful Health. Your body's largest organ has two basic layers, both of which need to be revitalized to give you the glow of youthful health. These are: (1) the *epidermis.* This is the outer, non-vascular, sensitive layer of cells that acts as a protective envelope. (2) *dermis.* This is the inner, true skin (also called the corium), which is composed of tough, elastic connective tissue with a rich network of blood vessels and nerves. It has an undulating surface, which is reflected in the noticeable ridges of the outer skin.

A revitalization program for the skin calls for opening the skin pores (which are microscopic openings in the skin) and sending nourishment and cleansing agents through the "tunnels" to the epidermis and dermis. This program feeds and rejuvenates the skin and results in a healthy glow that makes you look and feel alert and alive from head to toe. Throughout history, in all parts of the world, home remedies have evolved to successfully keep the skin healthy and young. These home remedies are as effective today as they have always been.

HOW TO BRUSH AWAY AGE LINES

Rose L. always had shiny, smooth skin. As a school crossing guard, her skin was assaulted by pollution from traffic, harsh weather, and tension. But Rose L. had an amazingly youthful skin that glowed with the radiance of good health. Many people said her skin was as youthful looking as the skin of the youngsters she helped across the street. Rose L. had learned to shield her skin against the ravages of the elements with a nightly "brushing" program. Here is the skin-rejuvenation program she used:

You Will Need: A natural-bristle complexion brush. Do *not* use a hairbrush or any synthetic bristle brush since it may irritate your skin. A pure soap, such as one of the many vegetable soaps available at cosmetic outlets and health food stores. A half cup of lukewarm water. A half cup of apple cider vinegar.

How to Brush Your Skin: Wet the complexion brush. Rub the soap against the bristles until you have a lather. Gently but firmly brush all parts of your face, throat, ears, and any other part of your skin that is exposed to the elements. Brush in a circular motion first, then brush up and down, and then brush right to left and left to right. Brush for at least fifteen minutes nightly. If necessary, use more soap for the lather. Keep brushing vigorously toward the end.

How to Wash Your Skin: Rinse the lather from your face, throat, ears, and other body parts with warm and then cold water. Be sure to rinse off every bit of soap. While your face is still wet (but free of soap), pour the half cup of apple cider vinegar in a basin of lukewarm water. Use this as your final rinse. Keep rinsing until your skin feels tingly and alive. Then pat yourself dry with a towel.

Benefits: This complexion brushing routine, as used by Rose L., has a unique benefit. The brushing opens up the pores of your skin surface. The bristles with the pure soap go deep within, scrubbing out the accumulations of debris that are sources of wrinkles and creases. The brushing cleans these pores, or channels, scrubbing the sebaceous glands, which secrete oily substances, so they can provide a regulated amount of youth-promoting moisture to the skin. Choked pores are frequently the forerunner of age lines and creases. Brushing helps cleanse pores so that needed moisture can replenish the "reservoirs" lying beneath the skin surface.

The apple cider vinegar splash is important because it restores the "acid mantle" to the skin. Basically, skin is acid. But most soaps are alkaline (except pure vegetable soaps) and strip away the protective acid covering. This leads to premature aging. With regular apple cider splashes, the acid mantle is restored, the pores are closed, and the skin takes on the glow of a child's skin.

Rose L. Has Roses in Her Cheeks. This nightly brushing put such a glow in her cheeks that Rose L. was often chided for having "roses in her cheeks." It was a well-deserved and flattering comment.

TEN SKIN-REVITALIZATION SECRETS FROM MILLION-DOLLAR BEAUTY SPAS

Skin-revitalization is an important program at some of the world's most famous and most expensive beauty and health spas. There is no need to go to these costly resorts (unless you enjoy being catered to) in order to undergo skin-revitalization. These beauty spas use a simple secret: *if it is good to eat, it is good for your skin, hair, and body.* All of these beauty spas use natural products that pamper and rejuvenate your skin. In just a few moments, you can give your skin a million-dollar revitalization treatment for only a few pennies.

Each of these ten skin-revitalization secrets will cost you ten cents or less! Try them.

1. *Skin Tone-Up.* Cut a cucumber into very thin slices. Massage slice after slice into your skin. The rich minerals will enter your pores and nourish the cells so that your skin will glow with youthful health.

2. *Wrinkle-Free Eyelids.* Put thin cucumber slices over your eye-

lids while you rest in bed. They will cool and relax your eyes. The vitamins and minerals in the cucumber are spurred by the enzymes to moisturize the lids and the surrounding region so that wrinkles are "plumped" and smoothed out. (Keep changing the slices as the moisture leaves the cucumber to enter your skin.)

3. *Smoothing Rough, Red Skin.* Cut a juicy tomato in half. Rub it all over skin that is rough and red. Let the mineral-rich juice become absorbed through your pores. Use the second half when the first half has been used up. Do not wash afterwards. Just towel dry. Minerals in the raw tomato will soothe inflamed tissues and help smooth out roughness.

4. *Wrinkle-Erasing Face Masque.* Beat one tomato and one raw egg together. Apply the mixture to your face and let it dry. Then wash your face with cool water. Pat it dry. The enzymes in the tomato take the vitamins and minerals in the tomato and combine them with the protein of the egg. Together with the fatty acids in the egg, they moisturize the skin. They provide nutrients to skin cells located beneath the surface. This nourishment helps counteract dryness and erase wrinkles.

5. *Hair-Thickening Shampoo.* Since hair is an outgrowth of your scalp, which is skin, it, too, can be revitalized and made to look thicker through natural methods. Beat an egg and use it as a shampoo. Rub it into your scalp. Wash out the egg with water to which you have added either lemon juice or apple cider vinegar to restore the acid mantle of your hair and scalp. The protein of the egg appears to thicken the hair shaft and nourish the scalp.

6. *Skin Softener.* Ordinary olive oil is a beauty treatment used at expensive spas to revitalize the skin. Massage pure olive oil into your skin. Keep rubbing until only a very light film remains. If possible, wear the oil film throughout the day so that its polyunsaturated fatty acids moisturize your skin cells all day to create youthful softness. You may also massage olive oil into your hair; then wrap your head in a towel that has been soaked in steaming hot water. Leave the towel on for 15 to 20 minutes. Then either towel dry your hair or shampoo it.

7. *Glowing, Fresh Skin.* Many expensive beauty spas have orchards of avocado trees. They need the avocado because it is one of their most effective skin rejuvenation secrets. You can use it at home. Just rub an avocado slice or avocado oil (squeeze it yourself or buy a small bottle at the health store) over your skin. Rub your skin gently until most of the avocado disappears. If possible, let the

avocado remain on your skin overnight. The rich emollient sub-stances in the avocado will moisturize your skin, nourish both the epidermis and dermis, and reward you with glowing, fresh skin.

8. *Beauty Bath.* Since your entire body is covered by skin, treat it to a "total beauty" revitalization program. Take a beauty bath. Mix two cups of vinegar with two cups of hot water. Add a few drops of your favorite scent if you like. Let the mixture cool. Draw a bath of tepid water. Pour in this mixture. Soak in it for at least 30 minutes. The vinegar will help replenish the vital "acid mantle" of your skin so that you will emerge looking and feeling silky smooth all over.

9. *Youthful Hair Sheen.* Boil a handful of fresh parsley in a cup of water. Let the mixture cool. Then rub it into your scalp and all over your hair. Wrap your head in a steaming towel. This will cause the scalp pores to open and admit the rich treasure of vitamins and minerals from the parsley to nourish your scalp. Then rinse your scalp and hair with cool water. When it is dry, brush your hair vigorously. Your hair will take on a youthful sheen.

10. *All-Natural Face Lift.* You can correct sagging skin, unsightly jowls, and an embarrassing double chin with a million-dollar beauty spa treatment at home for *under ten cents* and in *just 30 minutes.* Combine the following foods in a large bowl: one egg yolk, one tablespoon of dried skimmed milk, one tablespoon of fresh milk, one-half teaspoon of honey. Beat the mixture until very thick and smooth. Spread it carefully over your entire face, from your hairline to the hollow of your throat. Remember your eyelids and your ears. The mask should thickly coat your skin. Leave it on for about 25 minutes; then rinse it off with tepid water. *Benefit:* The amino acids in the egg yolk and the protein combine with the minerals in the milk and the vitamins in the honey to provide nourishment to your cells (which are made of protein), make your skin firm, and help smooth out wrinkles. The protein also revitalizes the dermis so that sagging skin can be "lifted" and made healthy again. In just 30 minutes, for less than ten cents, you can give yourself the same *All-Natural Face Lift* that is used by the million-dollar beauty spas . . . right in the privacy of your own home!

To rebuild your skin, treat it to a variety of these revitalization secrets. They will alert your body's recuperative responses to rejuve-nate your skin so that you will glow with health, inside and outside.

HOW TO STEAM-TREAT YOUR SKIN TO "ORGAN REBIRTH"

Like many factory workers, George K. worked in a chemically polluted environment. Day after day, his skin was assaulted by contaminants and poisons in and around the factory area. He had deep crease lines, chafed skin, unsightly enlarged pores, and a "hard-as rust" complexion. From his hairline to his shoulders, he had "sandpaper" skin that made him look much older than he was. His wife and family complained that he looked like he was in his 80's instead of his 50's. George K. was unable to cope with the comments on his rapid aging, so he decided to follow a nightly 25-minute program that the company doctor told him would rebuild and rejuvenate his skin.

The "Steam Treatment" That Rejuvenated George K. Every night, George K. would give himself a 25-minute "steam treatment" as follows:

Place a handful of herbal tea leaves in a large kettle. Pour in boiling water until the kettle is half full. Cover the kettle. Let the herbal tea leaves steep for three to five minutes.

Move the kettle to a table or countertop. (Be sure to put a burnproof mat beneath the kettle.) Remove the lid. Now place a large towel over your head and drape it, tent like, over the kettle to catch the steam.

Let the steam caress and envelop your entire face from your hairline down to your throat and, if possible, around your shoulders. The fragrant steam will open and cleanse your pores of accumulated toxic wastes and chemical contaminants.

"Steam treat" your skin for about 20 minutes. Then discard the tea. Splash refreshing cool water over your skin. Finish with a lemon juice rinse.

Benefits: In just 25 minutes, the nutrients in the herbs open up your skin pores and penetrate the epidermis. The steam helps loosen the accumulated toxic wastes so they can flake off. The steam sends the herbal nutrients through the pores into the deeper layers of the epidermis and then washes and nourishes the skin. It regenerates the sebaceous glands to restore a healthy condition. In effect, the herbal nutrients are *natural antibiotics.* They scour, cleanse, and disinfect the toxic waste-filled skin. The lemon juice rinse closes the pores to help protect against further poison infiltration. The acid in the lemon juice also helps restore the acid mantle of the skin, furthering improvement in skin texture and basic health.

From "Rust Face" to "Glamor Boy" in Ten Days. George K. followed this program for ten days. His entire skin underwent an amazing rejuvenation. His crease lines smoothed away. His chafed skin became clear. His pores tightened up and were almost invisible. His "rust face" and "sandpaper skin" took on a healthy, glowing, youthful texture. George K. changed so much that those who had chided him for being a "rust face" now complimented him for being a "glamor boy." Now George K. uses this all-natural easy "steam treatment" at least three times weekly.

HOW NATURAL AIDS SOLVE THE PROBLEM OF AGING SKIN

Nature is able to help solve the problem of aging skin. Following is an assortment of natural remedies that will correct defects in your skin. These remedies heal and revitalize your skin and help you turn back the hands of the clock so that you will enjoy an appearance of healthy youth.

Furrows, Sagging Skin. Combine one tablespoon of sour cream and one tablespoon of honey. Add whole grain flour until you have a paste. Spread this paste on your face wherever you see furrows or sagging skin. Leave it on for 25 minutes, then rinse it off with warm water. Finish with a cold water rinse. *Benefit:* The dairy fats in the sour cream are activated by the vitamins in the honey and the Vitamin E in the flour. They nourish your skin cells and even repair broken cells—the cause of much sagging skin.

Sallow Complexion. Combine one tablespoon of plain yogurt with one teaspoon of whole milk or cream. Spread the mixture over your entire face and throat. Leave it on for 25 minutes; then rinse it off with cold water. *Benefit:* The fermented milk of the yogurt combines with the dairy fat of the cream to activate your sluggish circulation, to boost the blood flow. The ferments contain beneficial substances that "wake up" delayed circulation to restore color to your face and brighten up your complexion.

Blackheads, Blemishes. Beat one raw egg white until it's fluffy. Add one teaspoon of honey. Spread this mixture over the skin covered by blackheads or blemishes. Leave it on for 20 minutes; then rinse it off with warm and then cool water. Blot your skin dry. *Benefit:* The pure protein of the egg white is energized by the vitamins in the honey. The protein then nourishes the sebaceous glands so that they secrete healthy sebum, which washes away debris from your pores. The protein becomes part of the skin cell structure and eliminates unsightly blemishes.

Wrinkles, Crease Lines. Add sea salt or kelp to warm water until the mixture feels gritty. Steam your face for two to three minutes to open up the pores. Then apply this mixture to your face. Rub it in wherever you see wrinkles or crease lines. Leave it on for 20 minutes. (Lie down and relax while this rejuvenation therapy works.) Then rinse it off with warm and then cold water. *Benefit:* Sea salt is a prime source of more than 20 ocean minerals as well as vitamins. These minerals help restore the fluid balance in the cells beneath the skin surface and thereby "cushion" the epidermis. By "plumping" up the dermis, the minerals make the epidermis firm and smooth. This treatment helps eliminate unnecessary wrinkles and crease lines.

Oily Skin. Oil attracts dirt like a magnet, so try this two-step natural aid. Use a pure, pH balanced soap and a complexion brush to gently dislodge the oil and grime from your pores. Then rinse your skin with water to which you have added lemon juice or apple cider vinegar. *Benefit:* The complexion brush digs deep into the pores to cleanse the openings and extricate grime. The juice or vinegar rinse disinfects the pores, and helps restore the "acid mantle" that is compatible with youthful skin. Repeat this treatment often until the condition clears up.

Dry Skin. Try a citrus juice face wash! Rub lemon juice, pineapple juice, or orange juice on your face. This will clean your pores and ease dryness. *Benefit:* The Vitamin C is seized by the enzymes of the fruit and used to repair the collagen, or "cement," out of which the connective tissues of the skin cells are made. Strong skin cells mean healthy skin.

Aged, Dry Skin. Combine one egg, one teaspoon of olive oil, and one-half teaspoon of lemon juice. Spread this mixture over the dry skin area. Leave it on for 30 minutes. Notice how it is absorbed by your thirsty skin cells. They "drink up" this mixture. Finish with a warm and then cool water rinse. *Benefit:* The protein and fatty acids in the egg join with the lubricating polyunsaturates in the oil and become energized by the enzymes in the lemon juice. They penetrate the cells and act as a reservoir of liquids to quench the thirst of the dried cells. Once the cells can drink fully, they moisturize the skin. Various glands within the epidermis spread this moisture throughout the body to counteract dryness.

Crow's Feet. Apply a thin film of baby oil and leave it on throughout the day and overnight. Wear this thin film regularly until the lines smooth out. *Benefit:* Baby oil consists of pure emollients that help to moisturize the dried skin cells and make your skin smooth and soft . . . just as it does for a baby!

Use these natural aids regularly to give your skin the look and feel of youth.

THE GREEK SKIN TREATMENT THAT TURNS BACK THE AGING CLOCK

While travelling throughout the Mediterranean, Martha E. marvelled at the youthful skin texture of the women in the area. In particular, the women of Greece had beautifully soft skin, even though they were exposed to the harsh Mediterranean sun and the strong winds of the mountains. What was their secret? Martha E. asked one Greek woman who admitted to being over 60 but had the skin of a teenager. The Greek woman told Martha E. about the ancient remedy that helped turn back the aging clock and keep skin soft.

Cleansing Grains Restore, Preserve, and Revitalize Skin. For centuries, the lovely women of Greece have used cleansing grains. Take a small handful of oatmeal (it should be ground very fine) and moisten it with water. Scrub your entire face and elsewhere for about 15 minutes. Then rinse your face with cool water.

Bonus Skin Revitalizing Treatment: Massage a small amount of olive oil into the skin. Leave it on throughout the day. At night, rinse it off with warm and then cool water. Pat your skin dry.

Martha E. Uses Greek Skin Treatment. It sounded too simple to be true, but Martha E. decided to use this Greek skin treatment. She had a sagging skin, "age blotches," and deep furrows. So she gave herself a cleansing-grain scrub three times daily. Then she left on an olive oil film for most of the day. She followed this two-step program for one week. At the end of a week, she looked as if she had had a face lift! Her skin had firmed up. Gone were the discolorations. Gone were the deep furrows. Martha E. looked 20 years younger. Back home, she uses this program regularly. She is deeply grateful to the Greek woman for this secret of perpetual youth!

Benefit: The scrubbing action of the oatmeal dislodges accumulated wastes and grit from the epidermis. Once the debris has been removed, the olive oil is able to quench the thirst of the cells and create a reservoir of moisture (key to youthful skin) that feeds the oil glands. This helps ease and erase age lines and restore the skin to glowing youth!

A SKIN-FEEDING PROGRAM FOR YOUTHFUL REVITALIZATION

The foods you eat are needed to nourish your skin from within. For healing and revitalization of your skin, you need to feed it a balanced diet of essential nutrients and important foods. Here is a tasty skin-feeding program that will help give your metabolism the ingredients out of which a healthy skin (and body) can be created.

Oils for Lubrication. Use cold-pressed vegetable oils to introduce much-needed polyunsaturated fatty acids as well as vitamins and minerals to nourish your skin. Oils put a natural sheen on your skin. They help turn an aged skin into a "plump," youthful skin. Use these oils in cooking and as salad dressing. You may also mix two tablespoons of any vegetable oil with a glass of fruit juice, stir the mixture vigorously, and then drink it slowly. This mixture will help lubricate your digestive system and moisturize your skin cells.

Protein for Youthful Skin. Daily, feed yourself adequate protein. Good food sources include lean meats, eggs, dairy products, beans, peas, nuts, and seeds. Protein becomes metabolized into amino acids which enter into the components of your skin structure. Protein is food for your skin. Protein can help firm up your loose skin and give you a look of youthful alertness.

Raw Carbohydrates vs. Refined Carbohydrates. In breads and whole grains, as well as in fruits and vegetables, *raw carbohydrates* are helpful in boosting skin health. They send energy and oxygen to the living cells of your skin. So you need a supply of raw carbohydrates from whole grains and plant foods. Eliminate *refined carbohydrates,* which include cooked, processed, chemicalized cakes, pastries, pies, cookies, macaroni products, and packaged desserts, since these are devoid of most nutrients. Processed carbohydrates tend to "clump" together to become impediments in the system. They can contribute to flabby skin and muscles. For carbohydrates, select raw plant foods or cook them just enough to be tender and then eat them with a bit of oil for a dressing.

Raw Fruits and Vegetables. Eat these daily. Eat them as snacks. Eat them for desserts. Eat them as part of a main meal, too. They are prime sources of skin-feeding vitamins, minerals, and enzymes, and they supply minute amounts of the other nutrients, too. They provide moisture needed to lubricate the skin. Drink fruit and vegetable juices regularly. These are speedily assimilated by your system and become components of the cell structure that creates youthful and healthy skin.

Seeds and Nuts. These help build a healthy skin and body, too. They are prime sources of essential fatty acids, which serve to lubricate the cells and "cushion" the skin to make it firm. Eat a variety of seeds and nuts daily. Use them for snacks. Add them to soups, casseroles, and baked foods. In a blender, mix a handful of seeds and nuts with a liquid and enjoy a delicious skin-nourishing tonic. Add chopped seeds and nuts to raw salads, too. Seeds and nuts are essential to a healthy skin.

Treat your body's largest organ to a program of cleansing and nourishing, and your skin will glow with youthful health.

IN REVIEW

1. Rose L. was able to brush away her age lines and rejuvenate her skin with a simple program.

2. Solve problems of aging skin with the ten skin-rejuvenation secrets from million-dollar beauty spas around the world.

3. George K. was able to "steam-treat" his skin and change his "hard-as-rust" complexion to a "glamor boy" complexion.

4. Solve problems of furrows, sagging skin, sallow complexion, blemishes, oily, dry, or aging skin, and crow's feet with all-natural remedies.

5. Martha E. turned back her skin's "aging clock" with a simple Greek skin treatment.

6. Revitalize your skin with a nourishing program of healthful foods. Skin rejuvenation begins from within. Feed your skin from within with healthy foods that supply nutrients to your skin.

How to Lengthen and Strengthen Your Heart Line

3

Your heart is the master organ of your body. It is your life-giving "pump." With proper health care, you can help to lengthen and strengthen your heart line so that you will have many years of activity. Let's get acquainted with this master organ and see how simple adjustments in everyday living can add years of life to this "pump."

Heart Works Around the Clock. Your heart is about the size of a closed fist and is located in your chest between your lungs. Your heart contracts and dilates at an average rate of 72 times a minute. This adds up to about 100,000 times a day—nearly 40 million times a year. The work performed by your heart is the equivalent of the work you would perform if you lifted a 10-pound weight three feet off the floor twice a minute for a lifetime. Your heart is the one organ of your body that never rests, except for that split second between beats. Your heart pushes the equivalent of more than 4,000 gallons of blood through your vessels each day.

Heart Health Is Vital. Your heart must be healthy in order to continue its pumping around the clock, year in and year out. A healthy heart is a more efficient machine than any man-made engine. As a "master pump," this organ is like an automobile engine. Feed it properly, and it will keep your body machinery running at full speed for a long, long time. Deny your "master pump" important nutrients or feed it the wrong kind of nourishment, and it can falter, become clogged, and run down. You can help lengthen and strengthen your heart line and keep your engine running healthfully with an easy-to-follow eating program.

HOW TO ADD "NINE LIVES" TO YOUR "MASTER PUMP"

To add "nine lives" to your "master pump," you need to keep it "oiled" and free of "rust" by following a basic eating program. This was the choice given to Joseph C., who was told by a public health specialist that his poor eating habits were threatening the health of his heart. Joseph C. loved food, so he needed to make some adjustments. Following is a nine-part eating program that he followed to satisfy his taste for his favorite foods while adding "nine lives" to his heart.

I. Dairy Foods

Eat Freely: Low-fat, low-cholesterol skim milk, low-fat buttermilk, cottage cheese, and all low-fat cheeses. Read the labels.
Limit: High-fat milk products, sweet cream, sour cream, ice cream, fatty cheeses, and butter.

II. Eggs

Eat Freely: Egg white, which is basically a protein, albumen. Eat all you want.
Limit: Egg yolk, which is high in saturated or "hard" fat and cholesterol. Reduce your egg yolk intake to no more than two or three a week.

III. Meats

Eat Freely: Trimmed cuts of lean meat. Trim off all visible fat before you cook the meat. Eat moderate portions.
Limit: Fatty meats and processed meats.

IV. Poultry

Eat Freely: Lean chicken and turkey, particularly the white meat.
Limit: Poultry skin, duck, goose, and stewing hen.

V. Seafood

Eat Freely: Fresh seafood prepared without saturated fats such as butter.
Limit: Shellfish.

VI. Fruits and Vegetables

Eat Freely: All fresh fruits and vegetables, raw unless cooking is necessary.

Limit: Canned and frozen fruits and vegetables. Prepared salad dressing, which may be high in fat. Use instead dressings made of oil and vinegar, lemon juice, or honey.

VII. Bakery Products

Eat Freely: Baked goods made with oils and whole grain flours.
Limit: Cakes, cookies, crackers, pies, pastries, and doughnuts, which are made with highly saturated shortenings and fats.

VIII. Bread Products

Eat Freely: Whole grain bread products, natural cereals (use skim milk), and other bread products made with oils rather than solid shortenings.
Limit: Artificially preserved and chemicalized bread products.

IX. Oils and Spreads

Eat Freely: Free-flowing oils, which help lubricate the heart and keep it working efficiently.
Limit: Solid spreads such as butter and margarine (unless the labels say they are high in polyunsaturates), jellies, jams, and commercial nut butters (these usually contain solidifying agents) unless they are labelled as pure.
Heart Given "Nine Lives." Joseph C. was able to build this simple but tasty food program into his regular eating pattern and was told that his heart was actually given "nine lives." He could satisfy his taste buds and his appetite since this nine-step program allowed him to eat most of his favorite foods. He could actually eat his way to better heart health!

HOW TO CLEAN YOUR HEART ON A FAT AND CHOLESTEROL WATCHING PLAN

Keep your heart clean by limiting your intake of hard fats and high-cholesterol foods. To understand how the plan can help "scrub" your heart, let's get acquainted with two substances that can be unhealthy.

Saturated Fat: These are usually solid fat of animal origin; for example, the fats in meat, whole milk, cream, cheese, and butter. Saturated fats are those that are hard and require refrigeration. *Problem:* They tend to accumulate in the body and clog up the heart, thereby reducing its efficiency.

Cholesterol: A tasteless, odorless, white fatty alcohol found in all animal fats and animal oils, in egg yolks, and in dairy products. It does not dissolve in water. An elevated serum cholesterol level causes your heart to become "encrusted" so that it cannot pump efficiently.

Fat and Cholesterol Accumulation Is Risky. Your body may absorb and store too much fat and cholesterol from certain foods. Accumulation of fat and cholesterol is influenced by more than nutrition, however. Other factors that affect accumulation include hormones, emotions, age, and physical activities. All of these factors determine fat and cholesterol accumulation levels. If cholesterol levels in the blood are high over many years, the "master pump" is in trouble. The arteries (including the coronary arteries, which supply the heart muscle with blood and oxygen) become clogged, there may be a hardening of the arteries, and the heart cannot do its job.

Arteriosclerosis. Accumulated fat and cholesterol may lead to arteriosclerosis in which the artery walls are made thick and rough by fatty deposits. These deposits reduce the inside diameter of the arteries and thereby interfere with blood circulation. There is an irregular thickening of the inner walls of the arteries that conduct blood to the heart muscles. The inner walls of these arteries (the coronary arteries) become narrow, and the blood supply to the heart muscle is reduced. This poses a serious threat to the "master pump."

OFFICIAL U.S. GOVERNMENT LISTS OF FAT AND CHOLESTEROL FOOD COUNTS

It is important to know which foods are highest in fat and cholesterol. Following are two official U.S. Government lists of fat and cholesterol counts[1] for popular food items:

Amount of Fats in Some Popular Foods
(Percentages Do Not Equal 100 Percent)

Food	Total Fat	Unsaturated	Saturated
Salad and Cooking Oils			
Safflower	100	87	10

---

[1] *Fats in Food and Diet,* U.S. Department of Agriculture, Washington, D.C. Bulletin No. 361, 1976.

Amount of Fats in Some Popular Foods

Food	Total Fat	Unsaturated	Saturated
Sunflower	100	84	11
Corn	100	81	13
Cottonseed	100	71	23
Soybean	100	75	14
Sesame	100	80	14
Peanut	100	76	18
Olive	100	83	11
Coconut	100	6	80
Vegetable Fats— shortening	100	46	23
Margarines—First ingredient on label			
Safflower, Tub	80	66	11
Corn Oil, Tub	80	64	14
Soybean Oil, Tub	80	64	15
Corn Oil, Stick	80	62	15
Soybean Oil, Stick	80	65	15
Cottonseed, partially hydrogenated	80	65	16
Butter	81	29	46
Animal Fats			
Poultry	100	60	30
Beef, Lamb, Pork	100	50	45
Fish, Raw			
Salmon	9	6	2
Mackerel	13	7	5
Herring, Pacific	13	5	4
Tuna	5	3	2
Nuts			
Walnuts, English	64	50	4
Walnuts, Black	60	49	4
Brazil	67	49	13
Peanuts or Peanut Butter	51	39	9
Pecan	65	72	6
Egg Yolk	31	15	10
Avocado	16	9	3

Amount of Cholesterol in Some Popular Foods
(Listings Given in Ascending Order)

Food	Amount	Cholesterol
		Milligrams
Milk, skim, fluid, or reconstituted dry	1 cup	5
Cottage cheese, uncreamed	1/2 cup	7
Lard	1 tablespoon	12
Cream, light table	1 fluid ounce	20
Cottage cheese, creamed	1/2 cup	24
Cream, half and half	1/4 cup	26
Ice cream, regular, approximately 10% fat	1/2 cup	27
Cheese, cheddar	1 ounce	28
Milk, whole	1 cup	34
Butter	1 tablespoon	35
Oysters, salmon	3 ounces, cooked	40
Clams, halibut, tuna	3 ounces, cooked	55
Chicken, turkey, light meat	3 ounces, cooked	67
Beef, pork, lobster, chicken, turkey, dark meat	3 ounces, cooked	75
Lamb, veal, crab	3 ounces, cooked	85
Shrimp	3 ounces, cooked	130
Heart, beef	3 ounces, cooked	230
Egg	1 yolk or 1 egg	250
Liver, beef, calf, hog, lamb	3 ounces, cooked	370
Kidney	3 ounces, cooked	680
Brains	3 ounces, raw	more than 1700

Official U.S. Government Recommendations on Fat Intake. "Some advocates of moderation believe that 38 to 40 percent of the total calories from fat is a reasonable goal," says this official U.S. Government report.[2] "In most diets this reduction can be achieved by simply cutting down on the amount of visible or separable fat used. Some say that less than 35 percent of the total calories should be supplied by fat. This much reduction in fat intake is not difficult to achieve but requires some modification in food choices and methods of preparing food."

---

[2] *Fats in Food and Diet.*

Official U.S. Government Recommendation on Cholesterol Intake. "Ordinary diets are likely to supply 600 to 900 milligrams of cholesterol daily. A 'low-cholesterol' diet usually provides about 300 milligrams of cholesterol daily. Foods of plant origin—such as fruits, vegetables, cereal grains, legumes and nuts—do not contain cholesterol. They contain plant sterols, which have been shown to reduce blood cholesterol levels."

YOUR FAT-CONTROLLED, LOW-CHOLESTEROL EATING PLAN[3]

Alice R. wanted to safeguard her family's health through controlled fat and cholesterol intake. She wanted an eating plan that would satisfy the fussy tastes of her family of five (including herself), so she followed this tasty program prepared by a specialist from a local health group. She was able to boost the health of the hearts of her entire family while preparing many of their favorite foods.

Avoid These Foods

The following foods contain large amounts of saturated fat and/or cholesterol and tend to raise the cholesterol level of the blood.

1. Fatty cuts of beef, lamb, pork, and ham, including hamburger, prime ribs, luncheon meats, cold cuts, frankfurters, bacon, sausage, and spareribs.
2. Fat-rich dairy products such as fatty cheese, whole milk, ice cream, butter, cream, and whipped toppings.
3. Most commercially prepared cakes, pies, danish pastry, doughnuts, corn muffins, cookies, potato chips, and crackers.
4. Egg yolks, organ meats, and coconut.
5. Fried foods cooked in lard or solid shortenings.

Basic Eating Plan for Heart Health

1. Eat less of the foods listed above.
   a. Eat more fish, poultry, and lean meat. Limit your total meat intake to six to eight ounces, cooked weight, daily.

---

[3]*Parker Natural Health Bulletin,* West Nyack, New York 10994. Available by subscription. February 2, 1976, Vol. 6, No. 3.

b. Eat low-fat cheeses, skim milk, and margarine made from a polyunsaturated vegetable oil.

c. Try fresh fruit instead of a fat-rich dessert.

d. Limit egg yolks to two per week. (Egg whites need not be limited.)

e. Eat organ meats only once or twice a month, as a substitute for other meats.

2. Reduce the total amount of fat eaten.

3. Substitute some polyunsaturated oil, mayonnaise, or margarine listing liquid corn, safflower, cottonseed, or soybean oil as the first ingredient for some of the saturated (animal) fat you normally eat. Depending on how many calories you can afford, use one to four tablespoons daily.

4. Choose and balanced diet that includes such low-fat foods as leafy green and yellow vegetables, citrus fruits, and whole grain breads and cereals.

5. Maintain your ideal weight by controlling your total calorie intake. Overweight results from eating too much food and, usually, too much fat.

Foods to Use

These foods are low in saturated fat and cholesterol:

1. *Poultry and fish*

   a. Eat chicken, turkey, and Rock Cornish hens.

   b. Reduce the fat in poultry by removing the skin before you cook it.

   c. Eat fresh and salt water fish often.

2. *Lean cuts of beef, veal, and lamb*

   a. Trim fat off before you cook them.

   b. Buy meat with very little marbling.

   c. These are lean cuts of beef: sirloin steak, round steak, flank steak, beef fillet, top round, sirloin tip, and rump roast.

   d. Buy only extra lean ground beef for hamburger.

   e. Buy lean cuts of lamb, such as lamb leg chops or roast loin chops.

f. Most veal is a good choice since it is young beef and usually contains little marbling fat.

3. *Dairy products*

a. Eat low-fat cheeses; for example, farmer, pot, cottage, skim milk ricotta, and skim milk mozzarella cheeses.

b. Eat skim milk yogurt.

c. Drink skim milk, lowfat buttermilk, and 99% fat free milk.

d. Do not use most non-dairy milk and cream substitutes since they contain coconut oil, which is high in saturated fat. Check labels carefully and choose only those made from a polyunsaturated oil such as soybean oil.

4. *Fruits*

a. Include one serving of fruit high in Vitamin C, such as oranges, grapefruits, lemons, limes, tangerines, cantaloupes, and strawberries, every day.

5. *Legumes*

a. Legumes are dried peas, beans, and nuts.

b. Use these as meat substitutes or as meat extenders in soups, baked dishes, and salads.

c. Legumes are high in protein, low in fat, and contain *no* cholesterol.

6. *Grains*

a. Include whole grain breads, cereals, pasta, and brown rice. These are good sources of the Vitamin B complex, iron, and protein.

b. Bagels, English muffins, and Bialys can also be used.

7. *Vegetables*

a. Vegetables contain *no* fat or cholesterol and are low in calories.

b. They are a good source of Vitamin A, ascorbic acid, and minerals.

c. Include two or more servings of green or dark yellow vegetables in your diet every day.

d. Recommended methods of preparation: steamed, baked, in soup, or raw.

8. *Fats*

   a. Use polyunsaturated vegetable oils: safflower, corn, sesame, cottonseed, and soybean oils.

   b. Use margarines listing *liquid* vegetable oil in place of shortening in recipes. Vegetable shortenings are partially hydrogenated and contain less polyunsaturated oil.

9. *Desserts*

   a. Eat fresh fruit or fruit canned without sugar (helps to keep calories down).

   b. Eat cakes, pies, and cookies made with polyunsaturated fat in place of solid shortening.

   c. Eat cakes made from egg whites, such as angel food cake.

   d. Eat puddings made with skim milk.

   e. Try sherbet.

Results of Fat-Controlled, Low-Cholesterol Eating Plan. Alice R. and her family enjoyed a delicious variety of these foods. They reported lower fat and cholesterol counts. They lost weight. They became more alert. Their "master pumps" gave them a new lease on life! They gained all this through a *family eating plan* that they all enjoyed!

HOW TO BOOST HEART RHYTHM
THROUGH SALT-CONTROLLED FOOD PROGRAM

Whenever Gary F. ate his favorite salted, spiced, and seasoned foods, he experienced severe chest pains, heart palpitations, and shortness of breath. The problem was that Gary F. loved highly seasoned foods. He knew that they were unhealthy for his "master pump," but he could not resist his urge for strongly flavored foods. He knew that he had to make some changes. One evening, after devouring highly salted and spiced delicatessen foods, as well as salted nuts and sharp condiment-soaked cole slaw, Gary F. suffered such sharp chest pains that he had to be led to a couch, where he turned pale, started to tremble, and perspired profusely, while gasping for breath. It was this "warning" that motivated Gary F. to make a change in his eating habits. He was shown by an insurance doctor how he could enjoy foods on a salt-controlled program that would be good to his palate and his heart.

Salt Can Be Organ Damaging. Chemicalized salt, or sodium chloride, narrows the passageways of the small arteries leading into and out of the heart. Salt also whips up the action of the glands to cause imbalances that can be damaging to the heart. Salt causes a swelling in the walls of the arterioles, those tiny artieries that carry fresh, oxygenated blood to the farthest parts of the body.

Salt Causes Swelling. As the walls of these vessels swell, there is less room for the blood to squeeze through. Blood keeps being pumped into the swollen arteries, backs up, and creates hypertension, which punishes the heart. In addition to swelling the arterioles, an excess of salt causes retention of body fluid, which results in a greater volume of blood and further raises the blood pressure. The climax is a strain on the heart that causes choking, sputtering, palpitations, and shortness of breath. Salt is the enemy of a healthy heart!!

The Heart-Saving Salt-Controlled
Program That Saved Gary F.

Gary F. wanted to have his salt and taste it, too. So he was given a heart-saving salt-controlled program that would satisfy his urge for salt but be good to his heart at the same time.

Basic Program: Use a wide variety of herbs and spices that give the tang and bite of salt but are salt-free. Try these seasonings with these foods:

Beef: Marjoram, onion, sage, thyme, bay leaf, grape jelly, mushrooms, dried green peppers.

Lamb: Mint, garlic, rosemary, curry, and broiled pineapple rings.

Veal: Bay leaf, ginger, marjoram, curry, currant jelly, spiced apricots, and oregano.

Poultry: Paprika, mushrooms, thyme, sage, parsley, tarragon, and cranberry sauce.

Fish: Paprika, curry, bay leaf, lemon juice, mushrooms, marjoram, and green peppers.

Eggs: Paprika, green peppers, mushrooms, curry, onion, and parsley.

Vegetables: Lemon juice, marjoram, caraway seed, dill seed, unsalted butter with lemon and honey, thyme, mint, parsley, onion, rosemary, ginger, mace, basil, oregano, and garlic.

Gary F. Becomes a Label Reader. Gary F. needed to avoid salt in any form, so he read the labels on packaged items. He *avoided* any products that contained any of the following ingredients (which are high in salt): salt, baking powder, brine, sodium, monosodium glutamate, sodium benzoate, sodium bicarbonate, sodium sulfite, sodium hydroxide, and sodium cyclamate. Gary F. also avoided the use of salt in cooking and at the table.

Happy Heart, Easy Breathing, and Healthy Complexion. In just three weeks, Gary F. (who continued satisfying his urge for salt with salt-free herbs, spices, and vegetables) felt his heart beat normally. Gone were the painful chest constrictions, the frightening choking sensation, and the shortness of breath. Now he felt heart-happy. He breathed easily. His skin tone was good. He had given his "master pump" a much longer lifespan on a spicy but salt-free food plan!

HOW TO BE SWEET TO YOUR HEART
ON A SUGAR-CONTROLLED PROGRAM

Refined sugar straight from the sugar bowl or cooked into foods can be very bad for the heart. Sugar causes a rise in the level of triglycerides in the blood. These are fat-like substances that are stored in the bloodstream. It is believed that triglycerides can clog the arteries and precipitate weakness to the heart. Refined sugar raises triglyceride levels so that the metabolism of glucose, or blood sugar, is upset. This can change the behavior of blood platelets and cause blockages in the heart.

An upset heart can cause reduced energy, frequent fatigue, muscular tension, convulsions, speech difficulties, hypertension, profuse sweating, a pale complexion, and painful palpitations.

Sweets That Flatter the Heart: Replace refined sugar with honey, blackstrap molasses, rose hips powder, berry juices, sweet herbs and spices, such as anise and ginger, maple syrup, mint, vanilla, sesame, finely chopped apple puree, diced pears, mashed bananas, shredded coconut, and pineapple tidbits. All of these are deliciously sweet and flatter the heart and should be used in place of refined sugar in cooking and in flavoring. Be good to your heart, help prevent erratic beating, chest pains, choked breathing, and more serious symptoms. Use healthy sweets that are good to your heart and your lifeline.

HOW TO FEED OXYGEN TO YOUR HEART
FOR MORE EFFICIENT PUMPING

Ned M. was troubled with angina pectoris (chest pains) whenever he had to walk more than a few blocks and when he had to walk up a short flight of stairs. He paused every few steps to clutch his chest, and gasp for breath. Then he would continue on his way, in measured steps. Ned M. worried about his recurring chest pains and shortness of breath. He wanted to improve the health of his heart and was told by a nutrition scientist that he was oxygen-starved. Here is the simple program that Ned M. followed to feed oxygen to his heart so it could pump more efficiently:

Increase Walking Limits Daily. Every day Ned M. would walk one more block. The first day, he walked one block. The second day, he walked two blocks. Slowly, he increased his walking until he could enjoyably walk ten blocks each day.

Enjoy Any Non-Competitive Recreation. Swimming, bicycling, hiking, and jogging could be enjoyed since he felt no competitive urge. (Frequently, competition—the urge to win—causes tension.) Ned M. enjoyed a variety of these activities and felt his breathing capacity increase.

Walk Instead of Ride. Whenever possible, Ned M. planned to walk instead of ride. He would walk a few blocks to a destination instead of using his car or a bus. He would even walk up several flights of stairs as his endurance increased instead of using the elevator. All this helped oxygenate his body and heart.

Supervised Class Exercises. When he felt better, Ned M. joined a local physical fitness group and participated in supervised class exercises three times weekly. He was being remade into a new and healthy person.

Breathes Better, Looks Better, and Feels Wonderful. In a few weeks, Ned M. could breathe much better. His face glowed with good health. He felt wonderful all over. His "master pump" was given air. Ned M. was given a new lease on life, thanks to an oxygenation program that cost almost nothing.

Why Oxygen Is Healthy for Your Heart. Oxygen is used in large amounts by your heart muscle fibers to burn the fuel that enables your muscles to contract. Your hemoglobin (the red coloring matter of blood cells) needs oxygen in order to remain healthy and to protect you against ailments. Your heart sends oxygen to your bloodstream, where it is used to create combustion of fuel and give you needed energy. Your heart needs oxygen to pump blood throughout your body. Provide nourishing oxygen to your "master pump" and be rewarded with a longer and healthier life.

Control Weight and Avoid Tobacco and Alcohol. Lose excess weight. Do not burden your heart with excess weight. Avoid tobacco since nicotine tends to tighten the arterioles of the heart and may predispose you to angina pectoris and heart trouble. Avoid alcohol because it alerts myocardial (heart muscle) enzymes and creates adverse effects through acetal (a substance resulting from metabolized alcohol) formation. Eliminate these bad habits, and your heart will be grateful for it.

As the master organ of your body, your heart can be kept working at a healthy, efficient rate if you treat it well. Keep your heart pumping and you will enjoy an extended life!

SUMMARY

1. Add "nine lives" to your "master pump" with the easy-to-follow, basic heart-rejuvenation program.
2. Clean your heart on a fat and cholesterol watching plan. Note the official U.S. Government listings and recommendations about these two substances.
3. Alice R. extended her family's lifeline on a fat-controlled, low-cholesterol eating plan.
4. Boost the rhythm of your heart on a salt-controlled food program. Gary F. ended problems of chest pains, heart palpitations, and shortness of breath with this tasty program.
5. A sugar-controlled program is sweet to your heart.
6. Ned M. followed a simple oxygen-feeding plan that gave his heart the breath of life and ended his chest pains and wheezing.

How a Raw Food Program
Heals and Revitalizes
Your Digestive and Intestinal Organs

4

Nature gave you a set of healthy digestive and intestinal organs at birth. They were meant to keep you healthy throughout your lifetime. With proper health care, these organs will serve you well. But with excessive wear and tear and improper eating, these organs may become weak and lose the ability to keep you healthy and comfortable. To help restore these organs to full strength, you must nourish them and pamper them. You will then be rewarded with youthful digestive and intestinal systems that will make life wonderful again.

Let's take a closer look at your digestive and intestinal systems and then see how natural programs can heal, revitalize, and restore them to health.

DIGESTIVE ORGANS: GATEWAY TO
YOUTHFUL HEALTH

Digestion begins in the mouth, into which food is placed to be chewed and then swallowed. Food then goes through the esophagus, or food gullet. Then it is propelled into the stomach where gastric juices (enzymes) transform the food into nutrients that serve to repair, replenish, and revitalize your body. Healthy digestion will create a more potent supply of vitamins, minerals, amino acids, essential fatty acids, enzymes, and trace elements to enter into the construction of your body organs and systems. Digestive enzymes also send nutrients into the bloodstream which transports them to all parts of your body to perform repair work and rejuvenation to keep you looking and feeling alert and young.

A weak or inefficient digestive system will result in a general weakening of other body organs. Your digestive organs must work in harmony in order to provide you with good nourishment and a healthy body. Just like links in a chain, if one is broken, the entire network begins to collapse. A healthy and well-nourished set of digestive organs is the gateway to youthful health.

INTESTINAL ORGANS: THE FILTERS AND CLEANSERS OF YOUR BODY

Some three hours after food has been eaten, it passes into the intestines or bowels. You have a large and a small intestine. Digested food passes from one to the next. A portion of the large intestine is called the colon. This organ must be in efficient working condition in order to properly expel wastes. If foods cannot be properly digested and then are improperly expelled, there is an accumulation of toxic wastes, which can create irritation or even toxemia. Disorders of any of the organs of elimination can cause a general weakening and even breakdown of this system so that the body cannot be properly filtered or cleansed. Problems include sluggish organs, malfunctioning organs, and irregularity. Symptoms may include constipation, diarrhea, colitis, and general digestive upset.

Keep your digestive and intestinal organs in good health. They are your body's filters and cleansers and must be properly nourished and cared for. They will then reward you with youthful vitality.

Let us see how natural methods can heal and revitalize your digestive and intestinal organs.

RAW FOODS ARE NATURAL HEALERS FOR YOUR ORGANS

Fresh, raw foods contain potent vitamins, minerals, proteins, essential fatty acids, enzymes, and trace elements, which become building blocks for your digestive and intestinal organs. These building blocks are powerhouses of nutrition and might be weakened or destroyed through processing and chemicalization.

When you feed fresh, raw foods to your digestive and intestinal organs, your metabolism takes the important *living nutrients* and uses them to repair your cells and tissues, enrich your bloodstream, create a healthy acid-alkali balance, and energize your organs so that they can function smoothly. Raw foods can help heal these organs so that your entire system can become youthful and filled with vitality. With fresh, raw foods, you can chew and eat your way to healthier digestive and intestinal organs.

CREATE SPEEDY REGULARITY WITH AN EVERYDAY, TWO-CENT FOOD

James D. was troubled with irregularity and constipation. He felt sluggish. He felt bloated. This embarrassing condition made him feel "sour" so that he was gloomy and distressed. He had a sallow complexion and walked with a stooped gait.

Laxatives Worsen Condition. James D. tried a variety of different laxatives. Powders, candies, pills, liquids—they all caused diarrhea, which left him weaker than before. James D. found that these laxatives became habit forming so that he felt addicted to them. Furthermore, the diarrhea drained his body of vital nutrients so that his health declined. He developed allergic reactions, frequent headaches, and general weakness. James D. wanted a natural way to strengthen his digestive and intestinal organs. He found it in an everyday, two-cent food that revitalized his organs so that he conquered the problem of irregularity.

The Everyday Two-Cent Food That Rebuilds Organs. This everyday food is *bran.* Bran is the indigestible outer layer of the wheat kernel and the husk of such whole grains as rye, oats, corn, and brown rice. It is also known as *fiber.* Bran, or fiber, is available at many health food stores at a nominal cost. It costs only two cents a day to put some bran in your diet. It is all natural, a healthy way to create bulk so that regularity is restored and the digestive and intestinal organs will work efficiently. A nutrition lecturer outlined a simple program for James D. to follow.

James D. used about two tablespoons of bran with his breakfast cereal every morning. He used another two tablespoons with his noon meal. He added it to soup or a vegetable broth, mixed it with a vegetable juice, or even baked it in a casserole or meat loaf. In the evening, he used another two tablespoons in chowder, as a coating for broiled or baked fish, or in any main dish. That was the basis of his simple organ-restoration program.

Boosts Raw Food Intake. Daily, James D. would eat an assortment of raw fruits and vegetables. These are good sources of cellulose—indigestible fiber that creates healthy bulk.

Becomes Regular and Bounces Back to Youthful Health. Within a short time, James D. experienced a feeling of over-all vitality. He became regular. He overcame his feelings of being sluggish, bloated, and "sour." His complexion perked up. He had the energy of a much younger man. His digestive and intestinal organs had been revitalized through this simple two-cent food, bran, and they rewarded him with youthful health.

HOW BRAN REBUILDS YOUR DIGESTIVE AND ELIMINATIVE ORGANS

Basically, bran is the coat of the seed of the cereal grain, which is separated from the flour, or meal, by sifting, or bolting. This is a machine process that passes the wheat kernel or grain seed through fine-meshed cloth. Bran is also known as cellulose, fiber, and roughage.

Cleanses Organs. Bran acts as an eliminator, scouring the mucous membranes of the digestive and eliminative organs, and helps to produce natural peristalsis.

Creates Natural Regularity. Bran contains a supply of minerals and cellulose that stimulate the musculo-nervous mechanism of the intestine. This increases the propulsive force that is needed for disposal of waste.

Provides Needed Moisture. Bran is hygroscopic in that it keeps moisture in your intestinal waste. This moisture provides lubrication to help correct blockage.

Soothes Spasms and Irritations. If you are troubled with spastic irritation of the intestines, the soothing, bland, demulcent qualities of bran will help relax the spasms, soothe irritation, and establish regularity.

Supplies Natural Bulk. The sponge-like quality of bran helps it expand with liquids to form natural bulk. This helps stimulate muscular activity so that healthy and normal regularity is created.

Repairs Organ Nerves. Bran also offers minerals and enzymes that offer a double benefit in that they will both stimulate and repair the nerves of the organs of the digestive and eliminative system so that there is better self-direction and the organs can work more efficiently for regularity.

To help establish regularity and repair and revitalize the digestive and intestinal organs, bran is an all-natural, raw food that should be enjoyed daily.

How to Use Bran for Digestive and Intestinal Organ Revitalization

Begin slowly. Plan to take from one spoonful daily to three tablespoons three times daily. Here is how to use bran:

- Use a teaspoon of bran stirred in a cup of yogurt.
- Sprinkle bran onto freshly baked potatoes.
- When making waffles, biscuits, muffins, and pancakes, add some bran into the dry ingredients before adding liquid.
- Add bran to meat loaf.
- Sprinkle bran over a raw fruit or vegetable salad.
- Stir bran into any fruit or vegetable beverage.
- Add bran to any whole grain cereal with milk and fruit.

Bran Is Most Effective When Taken With Liquids

Bran has the ability to absorb many times its own weight in water. The consistency of water-swollen bran is like that of a sponge. This helps create natural bulk and establishes regularity. When you take bran with any liquid (juice, milk, soup, and in cereal), you help enlarge and "swell up" the bran. This helps create revitalization of the digestive and intestinal canal.

Plan now to nourish your organs with healthy bran daily for revitalization and regularity.

HOW TO SOOTHE DIARRHEA WITH RAW FOODS

A much-abused colon (large bowel or intestine extending to the rectum) can react in distressing diarrhea or "loose bowels." Muscles of the colon become spastic because of wear and tear and general abuse, and they will no longer function healthfully. The symptom is frequent or excessive bowel movements.

The Raw Fruit That Corrected Diarrhea. Barbara N. was embarrassed by recurring diarrhea. Patent remedies gave her an upset stomach and worsened her condition. They gave her some relief from diarrhea but then gave her constipation! Barbara N. had abused her colon through too great an intake of cooked, processed, and devitalized foods. Now she was paying the penalty with an ailing colon. A registered nurse told her that she would have to follow a simple raw fruit program that would help repair and revitalize her colon:

1. Begin each meal with three raw bananas.
2. Whenever you want to eat something, eat a banana.
3. As a nighttime snack, eat a banana sprinkled with a bit of cinnamon or honey.

Benefits: The banana contains fine, fibrous cellular materials that are energized by its high mineral content. These materials then soothe and control the action of muscles in the colon. They work to bind and knit the broken cells so that tissue regeneration occurs to repair and revitalize the colon.

Diarreha Corrected, Feels More Regular. Barbara N. not only ate bananas as outlined, she started to eat more fresh, raw foods in place of canned or processed items. Slowly, her digestive system was soothed, and gradually her diarrhea subsided. She became regular. She is able to protect against further diarrhea with a more healthful food program. She has one simple rule: *Eat any food raw if it can be eaten raw; cook only what must be cooked.* And, of course, eat several bananas before each meal. On an empty stomach, the soothing ingredients of the banana calmed the frazzled colonic nerves, pampered them, and helped establish better regularity. Barbara N. feels revitalized all over!

HOW AN EVERYDAY GRAIN FOOD SOOTHES AND CORRECTS DIVERTICULOSIS

What is it? Diverticulosis is an ailment of the large bowel (colon) in which small pouches (diverticula) on its inner surface become packed with wastes and then become irritated and inflamed, sometimes causing abscesses.

Ordinarily, these small pouches, or diverticula, do not cause much difficulty. But when food particles become lodged in these small sacs along with bacteria, inflammation may result, which causes diverticulosis.

What Is the Basic Underlying Cause? Lack of sufficient roughage forces the muscles of the colon to contract with punishing vigor to create pressure that will move waste matter out of the body.

The less roughage in your body, the greater the intensity of the contractions in the colon. These contractions cause tremendous pressure. Often, the bowel is incapable of coping with this pressure. The bowel lining may burst through the surrounding muscles and form a balloon, or diverticulum. Neglected, these diverticula increase and cause diverticulosis.

Everyday Raw Grain Creates Relief. Ordinary wheat germ, available in almost any supermarket, grocery store, or health store, is the everyday raw grain food that can help nourish your colon and guard against diverticulosis, among other ailments.

Wheat germ is the essential part of the wheat kernel. This "wheat heart," as it is often called, is removed in the milling of white flour and refined cereals. That is why many diets are lacking in wheat germ. It is a prime source of protein, iron, vitamins, and minerals. These are taken up by your digestive system and used to nourish the colon. Most important, bulk is created, which eases and provides relief for diverticulosis.

The Healing Power of Raw Wheat Germ. Bulk-creating wheat germ takes the pressure off the narrow sigmoid colon (that segment of the colon which leads directly into the rectum). This bulk-creating substance acts as an energizer to encourage intestinal muscles to contract with normal muscular force. This helps reduce and even elminate the risk of bursting the bowel lining. Consequently, there is a soothing and healing of this lining and "pouches" can subside or even be eliminated.

How to Feed Wheat Germ to Your Digestive and Intestinal Organs

Guard against diverticulosis with a raw wheat germ program. Here are a few ideas:

- Mix about one tablespoon of wheat germ with two eggs for scrambling. Also add it to eggs for omelets.
- Garnish fresh fruits with wheat germ. Add yogurt as a flavorful topping.
- Add two tablespoons of wheat germ to one cup of applesauce.
- Mix two tablespoons of raw wheat germ into one eight-ounce cup of plain or flavored yogurt.
- Mix in a blender one and a half cups of skim milk, three tablespoons of wheat germ, one quartered banana, and two table-

spoons of pure peanut butter. Blend for 30 seconds. If you want, chill the mixture slightly before you drink it.

- Sprinkle wheat germ over any raw fruit or vegetable salad.
- Combine wheat germ with some polyunsaturated oil and a little apple cider vinegar for a healthy salad dressing.

Help revitalize your intestinal organs and guard against diverticulosis or "spastic colon" with raw wheat germ taken daily.

HOW RAW APPLES REPAIR AND REVITALIZE THE DIGESTIVE ORGANS

Peter O. had suffered for years from troubled digestion. He had recurring bouts of constipation followed by diarrhea. At times, he developed such painful stomach cramps that he could barely eat. He was nauseous at times so that he could not even eat simple foods. Peter O. had a history of eating cooked, devitalized, and processed foods. So he knew he had to make an adjustment. When his digestive system kept him up at all hours of the night demanding care, he decided to follow the advice of others who had recovered from such distress. Here is the simple but effective digestive-repair program he followed:

Breakfast: Fresh, raw apples—sliced, chopped, or as applesauce— with a sprinkle of wheat germ and bran and a bit of honey for flavoring. A glass of apple juice for a beverage.

Luncheon: Sliced applies with very mild cheese or yogurt for a topping. A glass of apple juice for a beverage.

Dinner: Assorted fresh, raw fruits, with chopped or diced apples with a honey topping. Yogurt with raw wheat germ and bran.

Benefits: This everyday fruit, raw apple, provides bulk for proper functioning of the digestive organs. Raw apple contains pectin and a natural form of hemicellulose together with a nature-balanced acid-alkaline ratio. These create an enzymatic action whereby the body's nutrients are taken up and used to repair and revitalize the delicate tissues of the colon and related organs of digestion. The combination of pectin and hemicellulose work to "coat" the intestine and send vitamins and minerals to the muscular network so that the colon becomes revitalized.

When the digestive system is given relief from devitalized, cooked foods, it can recuperate and regenerate itself to provide better health.

Raw Food Program With Raw Apples Creates Digestive Rejuvenation. Peter O. replaced cooked, processed, and chemicalized foods with fresh, raw foods. Whenever possible, he would eat raw foods and would eat cooked foods only if they could not be eaten raw. But he would eat raw apples with each of his three daily meals. When sliced, diced, chopped, or in applesauce, the apples tasted different each time. This easy and tasty program helped his digestive system recuperate, self-renew, and self-cleanse so that soon he could say goodbye to his constipation, diarrhea, and cramps. He had an "apple happy" stomach that made him look and feel alive with youthful health!

HOME PROGRAMS FOR HEMORRHOID RELIEF

Digestive and intestinal irregularity often causes straining at the stool. This may cause hemorrhoids. Hemorrhoids are swollen or varicose veins located just outside, inside, and across the walls of the anus. They can increase, if the straining continues. They can become so irritating that surgery may be required.

Raw Foods Pamper Abused Organs. Fresh, raw foods can help pamper the digestive and intestinal regions and ease straining so that the abused organs can become healed. Raw foods provide necessary roughage so that a movement can be created with minimal or normal effort.

Low Roughage Creates Unhealthy Pressure. If there is low roughage, there is the tendency to use force during a movement. Raised pressure within the colon causes the muscles to contract with unhealthy force. Pressure on the veins passing through the pelvis causes a back-up of blood and may lead to the formation of hemorrhoids or distended veins.

Eat Sufficient Bulk Daily for Normal Movements. Here are suggestions for feeding your organs sufficient bulk so that there is an adequate stool that can be moved with normal pressure:

1. As often as possible, enjoy bran with whole grain cereals for adequate bulk.
2. Raw vegetables, or vegetables steamed slightly, offer you a good supply of roughage. A raw vegetable salad topped with yogurt and sprinkled with bran and wheat germ makes a good high-roughage meal-in-a-dish.

3. Add lots of fresh, chopped or sliced, raw vegetables to a bowl of soup.

4. Use bran or wheat germ with green pea soup.

5. Citrus fruits are good roughage sources. Peel oranges, grape-fruits, and tangerines, *but keep the fibrous membranes,* which are sources of roughage. Eat an assortment of the fruits daily for snacks or as desserts.

6. Eat yogurt regularly. It contains beneficial bacteria that activate the intestines to perform more efficiently.

Take away unnecessary pressure from your intestines by adding bulk from raw foods so that there is less distention of the anus veins and less risk of hemorrhoids.

How a Garlic Ointment Heals Hemorrhoids. Here is a folk rem-edy that reportedly heals hemorrhoids. Thoroughly blend equal amounts of garlic powder and lanolin. When the mixture is smoothly blended, apply it to the hemorrhoid region. Leave it on overnight or longer. *Benefit:* Garlic contains natural mustard oils and a combina-tion of antiseptic agents, which together help to shrink swollen hemorrhoid veins. Ethers in the garlic are potent and can penetrate the distended veins to help bring about the exudation of toxic wastes and a natural shrinking. The lanolin acts as an emollient and soothes the inflammation, while the ingredients in the garlic can create the revitalization needed to soothe hemorrhoids.

FERMENTED MILK PRODUCTS NOURISH ORGANS

Fermented milk is a raw food that is a prime source of ingredi-ents needed by your digestive and intestinal organs for self-healing and revitalization. In the form of yogurt, buttermilk, and acidophilus milk, these fermented milk products are raw foods that are able to nourish your digestive and intestinal organs to create better health and vigor.

How Fermented Milk Products Create Healing. Fermentation of milk is brought about by a beneficial bacteria known as *lactobacillus acidophilus* or *lactobacillus bulgaricus.* These bacteria work to enter the digestive and intestinal region. From this vantage point, they start to destroy and nullify the poisonous substances that would ordinarily act as a corrosive irritant. Fermented milk provides your organ with this friendly bacteria that has a purifying effect on the region. An antiseptic action cleanses and refreshes the region so that your organs can be nourished, healed, and revitalized.

Eat Fermented Milk Products Regularly. Plan to eat yogurt as often as possible to feed your digestive and intestinal region those important purifying substances. Drink buttermilk as another fermented milk product that contains large amounts of friendly substances. Acidophilus milk is available at many health stores and some supermarkets. It, too, is a good source of *lactobacillus acidophilus,* which is needed to replenish your organs and help them self-regenerate for better health.

FRESH RAW JUICES FOR YOUTHFUL ORGANS

Boost the action of your digestive and eliminative organs by nourishing them with fresh, raw juices. These are potent sources of enzymes. Enzymes promote or alter action without altering or changing themselves.

When you supply your organs with enzymes, these wonder workers supercharge the system and send a treasure of essential nutrients to the cells and tissues for rejuvenation.

Daily, plan to drink a variety of different fruit and vegetable juices. You will also be providing needed moisture to your organs so that there will be less abrasion as they function.

Raw juices are like "oils" to your body machinery. Keep your digestive and eliminative machine in good order through lubrication so that they will work smoothly.

A Simple Fresh, Raw Juice Plan: In the *morning,* drink one or two glasses of any fruit juice. At *noontime,* drink one or two glasses of any vegetable juice. At *dinnertime,* drink one or two glasses of any fruit juice. As a *nightcap,* drink one or two glasses of any vegetable juice. *Note:* Throughout this plan, you eat your regular meals but *emphasize* raw fruits, salads, and whole grain cereals as much as possible for more organ nourishment.

Healing and Revitalization Starts Within 30 Minutes. When you drink a raw fruit or vegetable juice, the healing and revitalization start within 30 minutes. The nutrients in the juices have been freed during the process of liquefaction. They become instantly available for your bloodstream. These nutrients are then transported to your digestive and intestinal organs, where they are put to work almost immediately for healing and revitalization.

You have probably experienced a burst of energy and alertness after drinking a raw fruit or vegetable juice. You now know that it is caused by the rapid assimilation of nutrients by your digestive and intestinal system.

Squeeze Your Own Juices. Obtain a juice extractor at any health store or housewares outlet. Squeeze fruits and vegetables at home for fresh and highly potent juices. You will also be able to enjoy a variety of combinations. If you must used canned or bottled juices, seek out those which contain no sugar or salt and are free of chemicals.

Rebuild your digestive and intestinal organs with fresh, raw foods. Your entire body will undergo a revitalization when these organs are vigorous, healthy, and youthful. It's easy with everyday raw foods that taste good as they rejuvenate your organs.

MAIN POINTS

1. Your digestive and intestinal organs are the gateways, filters, and cleansers of your body and can be nourished with raw foods.

2. James D. created speedy regularity with an everyday two-cent food.

3. Bran is the raw food that rebuilds your digestive and eliminative organs.

4. Barbara N. soothed embarrassing diarrhea with a simple everyday fruit program.

5. Correct problems of diverticulosis with an everyday grain food.

6. A delicious everyday fruit helped stop Peter O.'s constipation, diarrhea, and stomach cramps.

7. Relieve hemorrhoids by correcting irregularity with simple home programs.

8. Fermented milk products nourish and revitalize your internal organs.

9. Raw fruit and vegetable juices create regularity and basic digestive and intestinal rebirth.

How to Air Wash Your Lungs
For Youth-Revitalizing Oxygen

5

With each breath of oxygen your respiratory organs and entire body become bathed with healing and revitalizing elements. The way you breathe, the positions you maintain during special air-washing programs, and the rhythms you follow influence the healing and revitalization of your body organs. Proper inhalation will help build better health and resistance to respiratory ailments.

RESPIRATORY ORGANS: DEFENSE FILTERS
AGAINST DISORDERS

Your organs of breathing represent your body's defense filters against disorders. With each breath, you inhale and exhale about 500 cubic centimeters of air, or about 16 fluid ounces. With more vigorous activity, you may inhale and exhale as much as 4,000 cubic centimeters. Each minute, you breathe about ten times. It is automatic.

Your lungs (which are situated in your chest cavity) consist of millions of tiny sacs, called *alveoli*, which have very thin skins. These sacs are surrounded by the tiniest of blood vessels, known as *capillaries*. Blood returns from all of the body cells to your lungs, where it is dispersed into the capillaries. The blood has left its oxygen in the body cells and taken on carbon dioxide, a waste product of metabolism. The blood enters the tiny capillaries of the lungs, where it gives up its carbon dioxide and receives oxygen. The enriched blood pours out to bathe your millions of body cells with life-giving oxygen. Your blood also picks up the waste product carbon dioxide and prepares to dispose of it. Your respiratory organs become defense filters against disorders and ailments. Keep them in good health, and they will keep you free from respiratory problems.

HEAL COLDS NATURALLY WITH EASY BREATHING EXERCISES

Edna G. had a history of constant colds. The slightest chill in the air would bring on sniffles. She often suffered from hacking chest coughs, a running nose, and choking sensations because of stubborn cold infections. Edna G. tried patent medicines, but they made her dizzy, and sometimes nauseous. She needed a natural way to restore the health of her respiratory organs so that she could heal her colds and, more important, build a defense against future infections. She tried a set of simple and easy breathing exercises that helped her conquer a history of colds . . . permanently. These were described at a local physical fitness class demonstration she attended. Here is her cold-healing program:

Position: Lie down on your right side.

1. Breathe deeply, slowly and gently forcing air through the blocked nostril.
2. Hold the breath for a few seconds.
3. Breathe out slowly and fully, gently forcing air through the blocked nostril.
4. Continue this easy, rhythmic breathing until the nostril is open.

Position: Lie down on your left side.

1. Breathe deeply, slowly, and gently as air is forced through the blocked nostril. Focus attention on your blocked nostril.
2. Hold the breath for the count of five.
3. Slowly and fully exhale as you gently push air through the blocked nostril. Again, focus on the blocked nostril only.
4. Continue this rhythmic breathing until your second nostril is open.

Relieves Nasal Congestion, Soothes Cough, and Ends Sniffles. Edna G. followed this easy *ten-minute* inhalation program whenever she felt the onset of a cold. It worked to relieve her nasal congestion and soothe her hacking chest cough. It also helped end her embarrassing sniffle problem. Edna G. is confident that by building up her oxygenation levels, she will be able to enjoy freedom from colds forever!

Benefits: This simple breathing program introduced a fresh flow of nutrient-carrying oxygen to the starved organs of respiration. When the lungs received the enriched blood, it worked quickly to give the blood the waste product carbon dioxide along with infectious bacteria. Now the blood, propelled by breathing, carried these cold-causing germs out of the respiratory organs and eliminated them from the body. This all-natural program healed and revitalized the breathing organs and not only overcame the cold, but also helped build body resistance to recurring infections. It carried a double benefit, and it was completely natural and totally free!

HOW TO AIR-WASH AWAY COUGHING SPELLS

A dry, hacking cough is nature's reaction to air and moisture starved lungs. Your respiratory organs need a healthy supply of both oxygen and moisture. This is made possible through an air-washing program, as follows:

Boil water in a kettle. Remove the kettle from the stove and place it on a fireproof or burnproof mat. Now *sit* at a level slightly above the steam. Slowly breathe in through both nostrils. Keep your mouth closed during the inhalation. Then slowly breathe out *through your mouth.* Continue this *breathe-in-through-the-nose* and *breathe-out-through-the-mouth* procedure until the steam subsides from the kettle. Treat your breathing organs to at least five minutes of this program. You will soon feel the cough subsiding. It may also help protect against recurring coughs.

Benefits: The moisture-carrying oxygen has bathed the tiny lung sacs, or alveoli, with lubricating moisture. This eases the chafing and irritation of moisture-starved capillaries. When properly "oiled" with simple moisture, your breathing organs will feel comfortable and will not protest with loud coughs.

HOW TO DECONGEST AND OPEN THE STUFFED NASAL REGION

Leonard I. could hardly sleep at night because of disturbing nasal congestion. In damp weather, when there were abrupt climate changes, or even when he left a heated house for the chilly outdoors, Leonard I. would fall victim to nasal congestion that would linger for days and nights without end. He would toss and turn, unable to sleep because he was unable to breathe. He tried chemical decongestants, but they gave him relief for only a half hour. He might have resigned himself to his affliction if a friendly neighbor had not told him that he needed to "unblock" his congestion by sending oxygen to his breathing organs. By "air-washing" or "ventilating" his lungs, he could restore his nasal region to good health. Leonard I. followed an easy program that worked almost at once.

All-Natural Decongestant Program: Leonard I. found freedom from stubborn nasal congestion and blockage with this four-step air-washing program.

1. Breathe in through both nostrils as much as possible. Even if they are "completely stuffed" they can take in air. Take in as much breath as possible. Hold it for two seconds. Now close one nostril with a finger and breathe out through the open nostril. Do the best you can.

2. Continue to breathe in through both nostrils and out through the same nostril while keeping the other one closed with your finger. Do this until you feel it is opening up.

3. Reverse the procedure. Take in as much air as possible through both nostrils. Hold it for two seconds. Now close the first or "freed" nostril with your finger and breathe out through the other nostril. Do the best you can. Continue to do this until the second nostril is open.

4. If both nostrils are so congested that it is almost impossible to do these air-washing programs, then breathe in through your mouth and out through one nostril while the second is closed with a finger. You may have to use force. Continue doing this until you feel the passageway opening. Then go back to step one and follow the procedure.

Frees Congestion, Breathes Easily, and Enjoys Sleep. Leonard I. followed this easy *All-Natural Decongestant Program* about one hour before retiring. He found that it cleared his congestion so that he could breathe easily and enjoy well-deserved sleep. After a while, he found that the stubborn congestion was leaving his body. Soon, he was free of this problem and could enjoy better breathing around the clock, thanks to this program.

HOW TO STRENGTHEN ORGANS TO HELP CONQUER EMPHYSEMA

Emphysema is an ailment of the breathing organs in which the walls of the air sacs (alveoli) become stretched too thin and tend to break down. "Air pockets" soon appear in the lung tissue. The contractile power of the lungs becomes weakened by excessive stretching of the lungs. This ailment can cause a barrel-shaped chest if neglected. Emphysema occurs when swelling is caused by air trapped between the cell walls of any connective tissue. To help conquer the threat and distress of emphysema, the organs of breathing should be strengthened through air-washing.

Anti-Emphysema Organ-Revitalizing Program

Position: Sit comfortably.

Program: Inhale slowly through your nose. At the same time, slightly protrude your lower abdomen and then slowly retract it so that your ribs are lifted outwards and upwards. You need to fill your lungs *completely* with air, but *without* strain.

Hold the inhaled breath for a count of three.

Now EXHALE through your mouth *on a sustained OO.* Your lips should form the roundest possible O. Exhale slowly as much as you can, but *without* strain.

Repeat this procedure three times a day for 10 minutes. Slowly work up to four times a day for 15 minutes.

As you feel your breathing organs becoming stronger, you may follow the steps while standing up.

Benefits: This regular intake of oxygen tends to restore the flexibility of your thorax (chest from neck to abdomen) and revitalize the organs contained in this region. The program also revitalizes the diaphragm with regular energetic movements. Regular air exchange is therefore promoted so that air pockets can be opened up and there is better ventilation. The program helps conquer symptoms of emphysema. It also builds resistance to the problem. There is more rapid elimination of carbon dioxide and poisons. This creates overall healing and revitalization of the organs of breathing and builds better health.

HOW TO STRENGTHEN ORGANS TO HEAL ASTHMA

Marcia P. blamed her asthma on heredity. Her parents and close relatives had asthma and other respiratory allergies, so she was resigned to enduring her choking, wheezing, and stuffed nose. She went the "medicine route" and took one chemical after another with the result that she developed skin rashes and became so drowsy in midday that she would doze off while sewing. After she fell asleep behind the wheel of her car and narrowly averted an accident, Marcia P. realized she had to give up her medications. Her symptoms returned with greater severity, and her recurring asthmatic attack left her weak and exhausted. Often, she would awaken in the middle of the night, seized with a choking and coughing spell that grated her lungs and left her gasping for precious air. That was when she decided to try getting to the *cause* of her asthma and using natural methods to remove it so she would be free of symptoms.

Strengthen Respiration Organs to Resist Asthma. Marcia P. learned that much asthmatic distress can be traced to a weakness of the organs of respiration. This weakness causes faulty breathing habits. There is a loss of the mobility of the lower chest and consequently, the upper chest becomes overworked. Strengthening is aimed at training the abdominal muscles to assist the diaphragm in some of the work of breathing. This promotes better oxygenation of the respiratory organs and relieves asthmatic distress. Here is a program prepared by a physiotherapist that Marcia P. followed:

Lung-Washing Program for Asthmatic Freedom

1. Stand erect. Lift both heels as high as is comfortably possible and then lower heels to the floor in one second. Repeat 10 to 20 times.
2. Draw in your abdominal wall and then push it out again in one second. (This is similar to a belly dance.) Repeat 10 to 20 times.
3. Sit erect. Suck in air and then let it out. Repeat 10 to 20 times.

Note: The preceding three-step program calls for breathing in and out through your nose only!

Organ-Strengthening Benefit: When you breathe out, your chest is lowered and becomes narrower. Your abdominal muscles and organs start to contract. Your abdomen is pressed against your diaphragm, which is then lifted when you inhale. This rhythmic exercise strengthens the bronchial tubes, the lungs, and the accessory organs and helps build resistance to asthma-causing allergens.

Pressure Breathing Strengthens Organs. The respiratory organs can also be strengthened and revitalized by being oxygen-bathed and nourished through this easy *Pressure Breathing* program:

Breathe in through your nose. Lift your chest as you breathe. Now breathe out through tightly pressed lips as if you were trying to blow out a candle held at arm's length. Repeat 10 to 20 times.

This *Pressure Breathing* further strengthens and revitalizes the respiratory organs, building up their resistance to allergens.

Marcia P. Conquers Distress of Asthma. For a short time, Marcia P. followed this set of inhalation programs. She found that she could soon breathe easier and better. Slowly, her choking subsided. She no longer wheezed. She could breathe easily. Soon, her asthma was just a fading memory. When her relatives saw how she conquered asthma, they, too, decided that it was not always "inherited" and besieged her for her "secret" of organ revitalization!

With organ revitalization, you can discover freedom from asthma!

HOW INHALATION THERAPY CAN SOLVE BRONCHIAL PROBLEMS

Bronchitis is inflammation of the bronchial tubes. Bronchial tubes are branches of the windpipe (trachea) going into the lungs. The smaller branches are called bronchioles. All the branches together resemble a tree, known as the bronchial tree.

Sensitivity or a weakening of the organs of the bronchial tree may cause bronchitis. Bronchitis is characterized by repeated attacks of coughing. Unchecked, bronchitis can so weaken respiratory organs that other ailments may develop.

Bronchial Revitalization Method

Strengthen the organs of your bronchial system through an air-washing program that calls for revitalization and healing of its components. Here is this unique and effective *Bronchial Revitalization Method:*

Tummy Breathing Program. Lie flat on your back. Bend your knees, keeping your feet flat on the floor or bed. Fold your hands on your lower tummy or above your navel. Breathe deeply through your nose and at the same time let your tummy expand. Hold your breath for the count of three. Now breathe out through your nose and at the same time let your tummy sink completely. Do NOT let your chest move at all. All of the work should be done through your lower tummy. Always take deep breaths and exhale completely. Visualize your body "melting" as you inhale and exhale. Repeat these steps for ten minutes.

Revitalization Benefit: The deep breathing sends a rush of oxygen throughout your respiratory organs. Since your tummy expands and contracts, much of the healing oxygen remains in your respiratory organs. It is the same as when you apply an ointment to your skin and let it remain without washing it off. The oxygen remains in these organs to nourish the cells and tissues and build resistance to allergens for a much longer time than it does when you raise and lower your chest with breathing. This procedure helps nourish the respiratory organs and build resistance to bronchial troubles.

Heat-Inhalation Healer. Inhaling comfortably warm air boosts the production of red and white blood corpuscles, which are then transported to the bronchial organs to provide comfort and relaxation. *Heat Inhalation,* or breathing in warm air, causes a dilatation of the tubes of the bronchial organs, opening congested passageways, improving breathing, and helping to ease bronchial distress.

How to Do It: Create warm air with an electric heater, several light bulbs, a heated radiator, or any source of warmth. Place a towel over your head (tent-like) and then slowly breathe in and breathe out. You will feel warm, soothing air. It goes to all parts of your body, including your respiratory organs. Slowly, as your breathing organs become bathed in warm, calming air, there will be a feeling of overall contentment. Bronchial spasms will subside. Repeat this procedure for as long as is comfortable. Your bronchial organs will be soothed with this easy *Heat-Inhalation* program.

HOW TO EXERCISE YOUR RESPIRATORY ORGANS IN FIVE WAYS

Here is a set of five exercises that will revitalize your respiratory organs so they can cope with and overcome breathing disorders:

1. *Hum Breath.* Breathe in deeply. Then *hum* as you exhale. Repeat for up to ten minutes. *Healing Benefit:* The gentle vibration exercises your bronchial tubes, pharynx, and diaphragm and strengthens them so they can function more youthfully.

2. *Cat Breathing.* Watch a cat "back breathe." Cross both arms over your chest as you lie on the bed. Breathe in very deeply. Now breathe out. Repeat this ten times. *Healing Benefit:* Deep breathing in this position sends a flood of oxygen to the organs of your lower abdomen and your diaphragm. These organs are bathed in and revitalized with nutrients from the bloodstream and oxygen. Notice how a cat will breathe this way when reclining. You are using the same principle.

3. *Air Scrubber.* Either sitting or standing, breathe in deeply through your nose. Tighten your lips and press them close to your teeth. With only a slender opening between your lips, exhale forcefully in a series of short air bursts. Follow with a few regular in-and-out breaths. Repeat this procedure three times. *Healing Benefit:* Contraction and forceful exhalation tends to send rhythmic vibrations throughout the bronchial tubes and the lungs, strengthening them so they can function without distress. This exercise has a scrubbing effect; that is, you "air scrub" your bronchial organs and keep them clean and healthy.

4. *Walk 'n Breathe.* Start walking with a natural, even stride with your arms swinging comfortably at your sides. As you take the first five steps, *inhale.* As you take the next five steps, *exhale.* Keep this up for 15 minutes. *Healing Benefit:* Walking makes a greater demand upon your diaphragm, and to meet this challenge, increased breathing sends a supply of much-needed oxygen to the bronchial organs and the lungs. You can help clean out impurities through this inhalation program.

5. *Alternate Breathing Method.* This is a two-part exercise. Begin by sitting comfortably, with your back erect but not stiff.

   a. Close your right nostril with your right thumb. Slowly inhale through your left nostril to the count of five. Release your right nostril (but hold your breath). Close your left nostril with your left thumb. Exhale slowly and evenly through your right nostril. Repeat this procedure up to five times.

   b. Close your left nostril with your left thumb. Slowly inhale through your right nostril to the count of five. Release your left nostril (but hold your breath.) Close your right nostril with your right thumb. Exhale slowly and evenly through your left nostril. Repeat this procedure up to five times.

Healing Benefit: This breathing method refreshes the clogged regions of your respiratory organs. It is an alternate, "crosswinds" type of air-washing that balances and stabilizes the oxygen supply in the system. It helps clean the respiratory organs of accumulated debris and rejuvenate the air sacs so they can be energized into a condition of youthful health.

Heal and revitalize your respiratory organs and body with air-wash programs that will make you feel youthfully healthy from head to toe.

HOW A SIMPLE BREATHING HABIT CAN CORRECT RESPIRATORY ALLERGIES

Many people with respiratory problems have a bad habit—mouth breathing. By developing the good habit of nose breathing, they can relieve much respiratory allergic distress.

Mouth Breathing Weakens Organs. Mouth breathing sends unfiltered air, full of dust, pollutants, and corrosive elements, and very cold or very hot air into the respiratory organs. This causes wear and tear that will weaken respiratory organs and render them susceptible to ailments. Mouth breathing is unhealthy for your respiratory organs.

Nose Breathing Refreshes and Revitalizes Respiratory Organs. Your nostrils are lined with hairs that are adapted to filtering inhaled air. These hairs trap dust particles and pollutants, act as a screen against corrosive elements, and also regulate the temperature of inhaled air. Mucous membranes lining the nasal passages moisturize air. At the same time, nasal breathing alerts special respiratory glands to release substances that guard against infection. So heal and revitalize your respiratory organs by making a habit of nose breathing instead of mouth breathing. Nose breathing is a good habit that helps build youthful health.

HOW FINGER PRESSURE CAN CLEAR NASAL CONGESTION IN FIVE MINUTES

Ralph O' C. participated in local yoga classes to help release internal congestion. He was told of one ancient yoga method for clearing nasal congestion *in a matter of moments,* without any drugs.

If your *left* nostril is blocked, apply finger pressure in the central portion of your *right* armpit.

If your *right* nostril is blocked, apply finger pressure in the central portion of your *left* armpit.

Ralph O' C. practiced this simple yoga method and discovered that his lifelong problem of nasal congestion cleared up in just five minutes.

Healing and Revitalization Benefit: Gentle pressure on arteries and nerves in the armpit that are connected to respiratory nerves appears to free blockage. It is similar to using a suction cup on a clogged drainpipe. Press and then release. This acts as a "milking" of the accumulated wastes. It dislodges them and enables the respiratory system to wash them out through the pores. This helps bring healing and revitalization to the respiratory organs. Breathing is free from congestion . . . without drugs . . . in moments!

HOW TO "NUTRITIONALIZE" OXYGEN FOR IMPROVED ORGAN HEALTH

As you air-wash your respiratory organs, oxygen energizes the bloodstream. This river of life then transports nutrients to body organs and the rest of your system. You need to "nutritionalize" your oxygen to create better respiratory organ health. Here are some suggestions.

1. *Vitamin A.* Helps maintain moisture of mucous membranes, builds resistance to infection, and works with calcium and phosphorus for better mineral balance. *Food Sources:* Liver, fish liver oils, egg yolk, and dairy products. Available as carotene, which is converted into Vitamin A by your liver, in carrots, broccoli, sun-dried apricots, cantaloupe, and leafy green vegetables.

2. *Vitamin B Complex.* Effective against invading germs. Increases the number of red and white blood cells in the body, which go to your respiratory organs to act as a shield and barrier against infections and allergies. *Food Sources:* Whole grain foods, brewer's yeast, peanuts, seeds, wheat germ, bran, and brown rice.

3. *Vitamin C.* Builds and rebuilds repiratory organ cells and manufactures *collagen,* the "cement" that binds and repairs millions of disease-fighting cells in the respiratory organs and elsewhere. *Food Sources:* Grapefruits, oranges, lemons, tangerines, and limes.

4. *Minerals.* Maintain acid-alkaline balance of the bloodstream, which helps neutralize infectious germs. The enriched bloodstream flows through the respiratory organs to act as barriers against infection. *Food Sources:* Dairy products, greens, raisins, seafoods, fresh fruits, whole grains, and fresh vegetables.

5. *Protein.* Needed to strengthen and repair the skeletal structure. Needed by the membranes of the respiratory organs to build their cells and tissues and strengthen resistance to infections. *Food Sources:* Lean meats, fish, eggs, cheese, peas, beans, nuts, and whole grains.

Emphasize these healthful foods so that as you air-wash your respiratory organs you also feed them so that they become healed and revitalized to reward you with the youthful breath of life and health!

HIGHLIGHTS

1. Edna G. conquered a history of colds with a simple breathing program.

2. Air-wash away coughing spells with an easy moisturizing program.

3. Decongest and open a stuffed nasal region as Leonard I. did with an all-natural, four-step program.

4. Resist respiratory ailments with the Anti-Emphysema Organ-Revitalizing Program.

5. Marica P. used a three-step Lung-Washing Program for freedom from asthma.

6. Use inhalation therapy through a special Bronchial Revitalization Method to end bronchitis.

7. Ease bronchial distress with the Helio-Inhalation Healer.

8. Exercise your respiratory organs to enjoy youthful health through five easy programs.

9. A simple breathing habit can correct respiratory allergies.

10. Ralph O' C. used easy, yoga-like finger pressure to relieve his lifelong problem of nasal congestion . . . in just five minutes.

11. Five food groups can help "nutritionalize" your air-washed respiratory organs for greater health.

The Natural Way
To Improve Your Eyesight

6

The eyes are often the most neglected organs of the body. Like other organs, they require good care to function properly. With natural programs, you can help correct problems of poor vision, weakness, and eye aches. Let us get better acquainted with your organs of sight and see how they can be strengthened so they can serve you well.

How Your Eyes Work. When light strikes an object in your field of vision, the light rays are reflected from the object to your eyes. The rays pass through the *cornea,* the front window; the *aqueous,* the watery liquid behind the cornea; the *pupil,* the central opening in the colored iris; and the *lens.* The lens of your eye bends the light rays as they pass through it and focuses them on the *retina,* the flattened, rear, inner lining of the eye, which contains *optic nerve cells.* The lens functions much as a camera lens when it focuses light rays on a film. The retina relays the light ray image through the optic nerve to the brain. The optic nerve carries the "picture" to the brain which is where you really "see."

Your eye is like a camera. The chief difference is that in a camera the lens is moved back and forth to focus the image, whereas in the human eye the eye muscles have to change the shape of the lens. To see clearly, your eye muscles must be strengthened. As with muscles of any body organ, they require regular exercise and activation so they can function healthfully. You can follow these eye strengthening programs at home so that your sight organs will be strong and healthy.

ORTHOPTICS—NATURAL SIGHT-STRENGTHENING EXERCISES

Orthoptics is a series of natural exercises designed to strengthen the muscles of the sight organs and thereby improve basic vision. Its name is taken from the Greek words *ortho,* meaning "corrective," and *optikos,* meaning "to see", that is, correcting the ability to see. As reported,[1] eye exercises such as Orthoptics can help strengthen eye muscles so that the sight organs can be restored to greater efficency. Orthoptics may also help prevent the need for glasses.

Here is a set of all-natural sight-strengthening exercises and home healers based on Orthoptics that will help boost the health of your visual organs.

Sunning Technique

Sit in a comfortable, straight-backed chair. Place a lamp about three feet in front of you. Use an ordinary incandescent light of any strength. Remove your glasses (if you wear them) and close your eyes. Now turn your head slowly and rhythmically from side to side, halfway to each shoulder but no farther.

Note: Let the light soak into your closed eyes as your head passes through the glow. Begin doing this activity for only two minutes; then slowly increase to a total of ten minutes a day. When you feel experienced, move the lamp to within two feet of your chair. Enjoy sunning a few times daily. Several short sunning periods are better than a couple of long ones. For more serious sight weaknesses, sun for one or two minutes every hour if possible.

Healing and Revitalization Benefit: This Orthoptic practice of sunning alerts your retina and helps to guard against brain aging, because the retina transmits images to the brain, stimulates it, and keeps it functioning.

Palming Technique

Rub both hands together until they are warm. Sit in a comfortable, straight-backed chair. Place a cushion on your lap and rest both elbows on this cushion. Close both eyes. Relax your hands and cup your palms lightly over your eyes, keeping the sides of your

---

[1] *Parker Natural Health Bulletin,* West Nyack, New York 10994. Available by subscription. Vol. 5, No. 15, July 21, 1975.

hands against the sides of your nose. Your fingers should touch your forehead. There should be no pressure on your eyeballs. No light should reach your eyes. This procedure should be followed for just five minutes daily to help refresh the eyes.

Healing and Revitalization Benefit: The warm, gentle touch of your hands helps soothe the frequently overworked components of your sight organs, making them feel tranquil and comfortable. This rests and refreshes the retina and optic nerve so that the entire sight organ feels revitalized. Your eyes will then serve you better with clearer vision.

Eye-Swing Technique

Stand in the center of a room facing a window. (Your glasses are removed, or course.) Keep your feet apart and parallel. Swing your arms very loosely, keeping your nose pointed toward the window. Swing your entire body—head, shoulders, waist, and so on—to the right as you put pressure on your right foot. Lift your left heel at the same time. Reverse the process so that your entire body swings to the left as you put pressure on your left foot and raise your right heel off the floor.

Note: As you swing, move your eyes along the lines where the wall meets the ceiling. Then swing your eyes below, gaze out of the window, and look as far into the distance as possible. Do this activity for one minute three times daily.

Healing and Revitalization Benefit: This technique helps your eye muscles change focus, which accommodates and also loosens any constriction or tightness of the eye muscles. This helps make them more flexible and less strained. Sight is therefore improved.

The Domino Technique

On a table, stand 14 dominoes (each having no more than 12 dots) about one inch apart at face level. Seat yourself far enough away for the dots to be blurred. Close you eyes. Start breathing deeply in and out. Now open your eyes and gently visually draw a circle around the domino at the far left.

Note: Do NOT strain to focus on the dots. Just look at the borders of the domino.

Repeat this procedure six times. Then go to the next domino. By the time you have reached the sixth domino, the dots should be in better focus and your vision should be clearer. If it is still not clear enough, follow an additional step. Close both eyes, mentally visualizing the first domino and using "mind power" to make it seem clear. Then open your eyes. You should be able to see more clearly. Go from the first to the fourteenth domino to help focus your vision.

Healing and Revitalization Benefit: The opening and closing motions of this activity activate sluggish eye muscles. This activity is a gentle exercise that alerts the action of the lens and retina so that they can function with greater vigor.

The Card Technique

Using regular playing cards, pull out the spades with numbers. Tape these cards on the wall one inch apart at eye level. As with the domino program, sit far enough away for them to appear blurred. Close your eyes. Breathe deeply. Open your eyes. Gently draw a visual circle around the playing card on the far left. Repeat this procedure six times.

Healing and Revitalization Benefit: The swinging motion of your eyes exercises the muscles that rotate the eyes. This exercise boosts the efficiency of your sight organs and helps them focus better. In sight disorders, the focusing muscles become weak, lazy, and unhealthy because of lack of exercise. Therefore, these outlined techniques "wake up" your lazy sight organ muscles and strengthen them so that they can function better with improved vision.

Basic Program: Continue these activities for at least 30 days, alternating techniques. It has been reported that within a month there should be be an improvement in vision. After several months, the sight organs should be much stronger for better vision.

Woman Regains Sight. These Orthoptic exercises helped restore sight to a nearly blind woman, as reported in the *Parker Natural Health Bulletin.* The woman, aged 84, was almost totally blind after cataract operations. She could distinguish only between light and darkness. She followed these eye strengthening programs for six months because of her serious weakness. But soon she could read newspaper headlines and identify pictures. Eventually, she could read for short periods with the help of strong glasses. Before the Orthoptic program, she could hardly see anything at all.

The Orthoptic program is intended to strengthen the muscles and components of the eyes, helping them relax and become revitalized to create better vision.

FOR SIGHT ORGAN STRENGTH
USE INCANDESCENT LIGHTS

Light is good for your eyes, but the source of light should be as natural as possible. Indoors, try to live and work in an environment illuminated by incandescent light bulbs instead of the newer fluorescent lamps.

The flickering light of fluorescent lamps can be upsetting to your eyes. It also tends to upset your basic metabolism and the rate of assimilation of essential sight-feeding nutrients. Fluorescent lamps provide insufficient long-wave ultraviolet lights and emit yellow and red light in a ratio quite different from that present in sunlight or incandescent lamps. Prolonged exposure to this unnatural light tends to weaken the nerves and muscles of the sight organs and can have an adverse effect upon healthy vision.

Incandescent light bulbs emit light waves that duplicate those of the solar spectrum or the sun. They also give off small amounts of long-wave ultraviolet light, which is beneficial and soothing to eye muscles. They can help protect against worsening visual disorders.

HOW TO NOURISH YOUR VISION ORGANS

Just as other organs of your body require nourishment, so do your eyes. When adequate nutrition is received by your eyes, weakness and illness may be avoided or overcome. A report[2] issued by Arthur Alexander Knapp, M.D., suggests that sight weakness and even blindness could be prevented through the use of corrective nutrition. Dr. Knapp has reported success with the use of Vitamin D and calcium. He feels these two nutrients are prime sources of strength for the eyes. He reports successful healing of ailments with these nutrients.

Keratitis Corrected With Nutrition

Sight Problem: In older people, the cornea protrudes more than it should. Instead of having the shape of a flat curve, it becomes cone-shaped. This distorts the rays of light entering the eye and reduces vision. Severe conical shaping leaves little vision, and "legal

[2] "Prevention of Blindness," talk delivered at 1974 meeting of the International Academy of Preventive Medicine in Washington, D.C.

blindness" may occur. Ordinarily, a corneal transplant is the only way to restore sight.

Natural Healing and Revitalization: Dr. Knapp reports that in cases of keratoconus, there is a body deficiency of Vitamin D and calcium. He prescribed these two nutrients to patients with this problem. Within six months, there was a noticeable change. Every patient had improved eyesight, accompanied by a flattening of the cone. Dr. Knapp claims that deformation of the eyeball is a symptom of a deficiency disease of the entire body. Because of this deficiency, he says, blood vessels become too permeable, which causes an excess of fluid behind the cornea. It is the pressure of this fluid that causes the cornea to protrude, which gives it a conical shape. "Given sufficient Vitamin D and calcium," says Dr. Knapp, "The cornea loses fluid and actually shrinks." This may help do away with the need for a corneal transplant, which Dr. Knapp believes "is rarely indicated."

Myopia Overcome with Vitamin Therapy

Sight Problem: Also known as nearsightedness, myopia is a problem in which the eyes can focus on nearby objects but vision at a distance is blurred. Dr. Arthur Alexander Knapp says that myopia is caused by an excess of fluid in the eye, which causes increased pressure, leading to stretching of the organ fibers and consequent distortion of the vision.

Natural Healing and Revitalization: Dr. Knapp conducted research on "highly progressive myopes. They were fed supplements of Vitamin D and calcium. Over 50 percent of this rapidly progressive group whose myopia reasonably would be expected to progress rapidly, instead showed a decrease in their myopia or remained stationary. One third of this series registered a reduction in myopia." Dr. Knapp says that a healing and revitalization of the sight organs occurs when Vitamin D and calcium shrink the most prominent portion of the eyeball. There is internal shrinkage and a necessary "dehydration" of the eyeball, which becomes reduced in size. Administration of Vitamin D and calcium treats a fundamental cause of myopia, *mesenchymal hypoplasia,* and strengthens the corneas and the scleras, thus scientifically and correctly reducing myopia. Here, too, blindness caused by myopia is prevented.

Brightening Up Night Blindness

Sight Problem: Night blindness is an inability to adjust from bright lights to darkness with reasonable speed, resulting in poor vision in darkness. It can be traced to a problem of progressive inflammation of the retina, noted by infiltration of pigment into the inner layers of the retina. This leads to weakness of that vital organ of vision.

Natural Healing and Revitalization: When Vitamin D and calcium were given to people suffering from night blindness (also known as retinitis pigmentosa), "without exception, every patient improved," says Dr. Knapp. "Most of those treated were the very advanced type with markedly contracted fields and often poor central vision. Following therapy, the characteristic apple jelly optic nerve atrophy disappeared and hyperemia (better blood flow) supervened. Night sight improved, central vision was upgraded and there was a widening of the peripheral fields."

Healing Allergic Conjunctivitis

Sight Problem: Conjunctivitis is an irritation and sensitivity of the delicate mucous membrane that lines the eyelid and covers the front of the eyeball. Occasional conjunctival plaques may form and pose a hazard to eye health by causing an ulcer on the cornea. Untreated, it may destroy sight-making powers of the organ.

Natural Healing and Revitalization: "For years," says Dr. Knapp, "Vitamin D and calcium have been prescribed (for allergic conjunctivitis) and over 90 percent of the patients have improved. Complaints of sensitivity to light, itching and tearing usually disappear completely or improve markedly, though a few patients have an occasional mild exacerbation (flaring up). It may take two to three weeks for the desired local effect, dependent upon a changed systemic calcium balance."

Dr. Knapp's Recommendations: For treating disorders of the sight organs, Dr. Knapp recommends using 50,000 units a day of Vitamin D. "For the past 20 odd years, I have seen no toxicity from the intermittent daily administration of 50,000 units." As for calcium, he administers 1,000 milligrams per day. Both nutrients are taken orally.

Dr. Arthur Alexander Knapp claims to be able to heal these four basic sight organ disorders with two nutrients. These nutrients are effective in nourishing the components of the organs and thereby correct and overcome disorders and help bring newer, better, and, often, restored vision.

FOLK HEALERS FOR COMMON AND
UNCOMMON EYE DISORDERS

Heal and revitalize your eyes by correcting visual disorders with all-natural folk healers. These are especially beneficial in helping to ease reactions to air pollution and tired, burning, and itching eyes. These are symptoms of organ unrest, which can be soothed with folk healers.

Inflamed Eyes. Put one or two drops of fresh castor oil (be sure it is fresh and not rancid) in the eyes and on the eyelids. Burning sensations will be cooled, and the eyes will feel refreshed.

Tired, Itching Eyes. Boil three tablespoons of honey in two cups of water. When the honey is thoroughly dissolved, let the mixture cool. Then use the mixture as a natural eye wash several times throughout the day. TIP: For speedy healing, dip a pad of absorbent cotton into the healer and use it as an all-natural, soothing compress upon the eyes.

Tired Eyes. Help ease a "bloodshot" look by moistening herbal tea bags with boiling water. When the bags are comfortably cool, apply them as a compress to the eyes while you recline in a darkened room. Ingredients in the herbs appear to refresh the eyes and re-distribute the congested blood accumulation.

Inflammation, Sties in Eyes. Steam fresh cabbage leaves in boil-ing water. When they are limp but not cooked, remove them and drain them. Apply the warm leaves to your closed eyes. Relax on a couch or bed. Keep repeating this cabbage leaf application until the problems are gone.

Blurred Vision. Blurred vision is frequently a symptom of eye-strain. You can obtain relief by making a poultice out of grated raw potato and potato juice. Apply the poultice to the closed eyes as you relax in bed. Leave it on for up to 30 minutes. Keep renewing the poultice until your eyes feel better and your vision is clearer.

Basic Eye Health Revitalizer: Throughout the day, revitalize your tired eyes by resting regularly. Splash cold water over your eyes. Apply a cold wet compress for ten to fifteen minutes at frequent intervals. Close your eyes. Roll them to the far right, the far left, all the way up, and all the way down. Frequently, close your eyes and massage gently with one finger in a circular motion over your eyeball.

Let nature help heal and revitalize your organs of sight so that you can enjoy better vision.

FOUR WAYS TO FREE YOUR EYES FROM STRAIN

Bookkeeper Dorothy Q. was the victim of occupational eye strain. Having to add up long columns of figures gave Dorothy Q. such severe eye strain that her vision became blurred. She could not thread a needle, except at very close range. Her favorite pastime of reading now became painful. She wanted to free her eyes from strain and was given a simple four-step program by her optometrist that would help revitalize her muscles of sight:

1. Begin by closing your eyes. Take a short "eye vacation" to any soothing or comforting scene you can visualize. With closed eyes, "see" this peaceful scene and enjoy it.

2. Close your eyes. Now "see" something that is familiar, such as a garment, a painting, a friend's face, or favorite foods.

3. Open your eyes. Look at something nearby. It doesn't matter what the object is as long as you look at it fixedly. Now close your eyes. Cover them with your palms. Picture the same object. Visualize the shape, color, size, texture, location, and function of that object. "See" it as you did before, but with your eyes closed.

4. Open your eyes. Look at a soothing picture on the wall. Close your eyes and cover them with your palms. Visualize the picture. You may even project yourself into the picture. Visualize why the picture was created and what its message may be.

Just Five to Ten Minutes at a Time Soothes Eye Organs. Dorothy Q. spent less than ten minutes at a time doing this four-step sight revitalization program. It helped relax her eye muscles, refresh them, and relieve them of strain. After a few such sessions, Dorothy Q. felt her eyes becoming restored. Soon the ache was gone and her vision became more acute so that she could thread needles and read comfortably. Her sight organs and her entire being now became revitalized.

BLINKING IS A NATURAL EYEWASH

The burning, scratchy sensation in his eyes made Jimmy S. nervous and irritable. As a dairy farmer, he spent a lot of time in the barn, where he needed good eyesight to manage his machinery for milking. When Jimmy S. experienced burning and scratching eyes, he had to stop and close them until the feeling passed. But relief was temporary. To relieve his recurring burning, he tried chemical eye potions, but they further irritated his eyes. He needed a natural eyewash. He was told of one that cost *nothing* and was the best eyewash nature could offer.

Blinking Is Key to Eye Comfort. Jimmy S. was told by his eye specialist to blink frequently throughout the day. The blinking process is like "milking" the lacrimal glands (located at the side of each eyeball), which then shed tears. Blinking also activates the meibomian glands (small glands on the inner surface of the eyelids) to release an oily liquid that further lubricates the eyes. In other words, blinking stimulates the lacrimal and meibomian glands to wash away accumulated dust, pollution, wastes, and irritants.

Jimmy S. would pause as frequently as possible to blink and blink and blink away harsh irritants that were responsible for his burning and scratching. After a few days, his condition cleared up. Now, Jimmy S. is a contented dairy farmer with clear, bright eyes that are washed regularly with blinking!

HOW TO BE GOOD TO YOUR EYES

Reduce fatigue of eye muscles by reading in good light. A 100 watt bulb at a distance of four feet will provide sufficient illumination for close work. The entire room should be properly lit for good eye comfort. Your eyes will be less strained if the whole room is as bright as the region of focus. Use a light-colored desk or tabletop and walls since they will *reflect* light, which makes sight more comfortable. Restrict or eliminate dark-colored objects or walls since they *absorb* light and reduce eye comfort and efficiency. Protect your eyes against fatigue and strain by avoiding any darkened or improperly illuminated area.

When watching television, sit about ten feet away from the screen. Do not stare at the screen for more than ten minutes at a time. Regularly divert your visual attention and look around the room. This helps exercise the muscles of your eyes. Periodically cover both eyes with your palms and gently massage the eyeballs. This will help refresh your eyes and protect against congestion and sight disorders.

Be good to your eyes, and you will enjoy better vision, better body health, and a feeling of total revitalization that makes life worth living.

SUMMARY

1. Heal and revitalize your eye organs with Orthoptics, exercises that boost visual efficiency and health.
2. An 84-year-old woman, nearly blind after cataract operations, enjoyed sight restoration because of the Orthoptic program.
3. Correct sight problems such as keratitis, myopia (nearsightedness), night blindness, and allergic conjunctivitis with two nutrients, as recommended by a physician.
4. Inflamed, itchy, tired, and blurred eyes are restored and revitalized through natural folk healers.
5. Dorothy Q. freed her eyes from strain by following a four-step program.
6. Jimmy S. used blinking as a natural eyewash to correct burning and scratching of his eyes.
7. Be good to your eyes, and they will reward you with clear vision and basic body health.

Home Treatments to
Improve Your Organs of Hearing

7

Good hearing is important to provide you with a feeling of safety, success, and satisfaction. When your organs of hearing are in good health, you are able to enjoy life and participate in all of its pleasures. To better understand how to improve your organs of hearing, you should be acquainted with the components of your ears.

Basics About Your Hearing Organs. Your ear consists of three basic parts: the outer, middle, and inner ear. Your *outer* ear is a trumpet-shaped organ with a funnel, or duct, that extends into your ear drum. The ear drum is a thin, tightly stretched membrane that vibrates when sound waves strike it, like the top of a drum. Your *middle* ear is directly opposite your outer ear. It contains three small bones shaped respectively like a hammer, an anvil, and a stirrup. When sound waves cause the ear drum to vibrate, the vibration moves to these tiny bones and from there to the fluid of the *inner* ear. In the inner ear, microscopically small hairs waving back and forth conduct the vibration to the nerve of hearing, which transmits it electrically to your brain.

Eustachian Tube. Your middle ear is connected to your throat by the eustachian tube, which allows air to move in and out to equalize the atmospheric pressure. If your ear hurts at high altitudes, you can swallow to normalize the pressure through the eustachian tube and become comfortable again.

Inner Ear Organs. Still deeper in your head is your inner ear. One part, composed of three semi-circular canals, is the mechanism by which you balance your body. If this organ malfunctions, you may become dizzy or unable to maintain normal balance. The other part of your inner ear is shaped like a snail shell, so it is called the cockle shell or *cochlea*. In it, the nerve of hearing is spread out to catch sound impressions and carry them to your brain.

Your organs of hearing require proper nutritional and basic health care to be able to reward you with the ability to hear properly.

HOW A THREE-STEP FOOD PROGRAM RESTORED HEARING

A physician has reported that a three-step food program restored his formerly "lost" hearing.[1] An ear specialist himself, James T. Spencer, M.D., found that he was losing his hearing and suffering from recurring dizziness and vertigo. Dr. Spencer self-prescribed this three-step food program after undergoing several tests:

1. Eliminate all refined carbohydrates from meals.
2. Limit the amount of carbohydrates eaten.
3. Reduce the intake of saturated fats such as fatty meats, cream, butter, and fried foods.

Findings: Dr. Spencer says that his hearing loss could be traced to very high cholesterol and triglyceride readings in his bloodstream. These two fatty substances tend to constrict the arteries of the organs of hearing and are believed to create "blocks" that restrict the passage of sound waves.

Cholesterol is a fat-like substance found only in animal products. *Triglycerides,* fatty elements in the bloodstream, are a form of storage for excess carbohydrates eaten. Triglycerides formed from sugar are much more persistent than those formed from starch. They are not easily or quickly cleared out of the bloodstream. Too many triglycerides can clog the arteries involved in the organs of hearing and thus can contribute to the malfunctioning of hearing.

Hearing Regained and Health Restored. Dr. James T. Spencer reports that 90 days after he started this simple three-step program, his cholesterol and triglyceride levels were lower. He had lost 14 excess pounds. *He had regained nearly all of his "lost" hearing.* Because *saturated fats may cause hardening of the arteries affecting the ear and thereby create hearing loss,* a restriction of refined carbohydrates and hard fats can help protect against this type of hearing loss. Without such a diet, accumulated carbohydrates and hard fats may affect those delicate inner ear segments that regulate hearing acuity.

Patients Enjoy Better Hearing on Three-Step Food Plan. Dr.

[1] *Parker Natural Health Bulletin,* West Nyack, New York, 10994. Available by subscription. Vol 6, No. 16. August 2, 1976.

Spencer reports that his patients enjoyed improved hearing with this three-step food plan. One patient had suffered from hearing loss, vertigo, and ear ringing that he described as a "maddening roar." He was overweight. Tests showed he had a very high level of fat in the blood. After only 21 days on Dr. Spencer's three-step food plan, this man began to experience hearing restoration as well as a much-needed loss of weight. And the dizziness and ear ringing ended! Other patients also experienced a hearing recovery as well as general health improvement.

Basic Ear Organ Healer. Dr. Spencer's basic ear organ healing and revitalization plan consists of this simple three-step program; namely, eliminate refined carbohydrates, limit the amount of carbohydrates eaten, and reduce the intake of hard fats. This is the natural way to help restore hearing.

HOW NUTRITION IMPROVED HEALTH OF HEARING ORGANS

The *Parker Natural Health Bulletin* also refers to a program of vitamin therapy for patients at the Mayo Clinic. These patients were troubled with meniere's disease (an ear problem consisting of dizziness, nausea, inner ear disturbance, and progressive deafness). Doctors gave them daily doses of 600 milligrams of Vitamin C and 600 milligrams of bioflavonoids (nutrients that accompany Vitamin C) together with large amounts of B vitamins. They did *not* prescribe any special diets.

Hearing Restored, Problems Solved. On this vitamin program, nearly all patients experienced hearing restoration, while nausea, ear ringing, and vertigo gradually vanished. This simple nutritional vitamin program created healing and revitalization of the hearing organs.

High-Vitamin, Salt-Free Diet Leads to Hearing Improvement

The *Parker Natural Health Bulletin* tells of a supervised program in which doctors prescribed a high-vitamin, salt-free diet to help ease hearing disorders in their patients. They specifically prescribed niacin, one of the B-complex vitamins, because it acts as a vasodilator. It helps dilate blood vessels to permit more nourishment to travel to the cochlea so it can catch sounds efficiently and transport them to your brain. Patients took 25 milligrams of niacin twice daily, slowly increasing to 100 milligrams daily. Symptoms subsided gradually.

A salt-free diet was helpful because salt absorbs water in the tissues, which may cause inner ear disturbances.

Gradually, the hearing organs of the patients were strengthened, and they were free from the problems of hearing loss and progressive deafness.

EASY EXERCISES TO HELP YOU HEAR BETTER

Blocked Hearing. If sound waves are blocked and there is a reduction in transmission, try these easy exercises:

- Open the clogged ear portals by saying the following words aloud: *yee, air,* and *you.* Make a face to exaggerate these words in a long and loud tone. Repeat these words several times daily.

- Insert a wad of cotton or a clean compress behind your last tooth. Bite down very hard for a few moments. Repeat this procedure five times several times during the day.

- Gently press the fat pads of your middle fingertips in your ears. Now hum any gentle tune. Do this repeatedly throughout the day. The vibrations will help stimulate the small hairs of your inner ear and promote better hearing.

- Boost a congested circulation by loosening pockets of debris. Throughout the day, bend your head forward three times, backward three times, to your left three times, and to your right three times. This activity helps loosen tight joints and permits freer transportation of oxygen, blood, and nutrients to your ears.

How a Plant Food Program Restored Hearing

Phyllis X. was becoming worried about her slowly decreasing ability to hear. Friends and family had to shout to make themselves heard. Radio and television had to be turned on so loud that other family members had to leave the room. Phyllis X. feared progressive hearing loss. Rather than face a world of silence, she agreed to follow a very simple food program, prepared by her ear doctor, that would help restore hearing.

More Plant Foods, Fewer Animal Foods. Daily, Phyllix X. would eat more plant foods—fresh, raw and cooked fruits, vegetables, grains, beans, seeds, and nuts—and *fewer* animal foods. Soon she found that she could enjoy an almost complete plant food program with only an occasional meat dish to satisfy a special taste.

Hearing Is Gradually Restored. Phyllis X. found her hearing becoming more acute. She could hear better and better. Voices no longer had to be raised. Radio and television could be enjoyed at normal sound levels. When she experienced a total healing of her ear organs, she continued with her high-plant-food and low-animal-food program. She feels rescued from a world of silence.

Healing and Revitalization Benefit: In many older persons, there is a tendency for the arteries that feed the ears to become congested with accumulated cholesterol. A high-animal-food diet will deposit more cholesterol than the body can accommodate, which causes arterial constriction. Hearing can grow weak. On a low-cholesterol program, arteries are cleansed and can transport oxygen and nutrients to the ears. Narrowed or "cholesterol-choked" arteries may dull hearing by blocking flow to the cochlea, the shell-shaped organ within the skull which houses auditory nerve endings. By going on a cholesterol-controlled eating program, with less emphasis on animal foods and more emphasis on plant foods, you can rejuvenate your arteries and make them more resilient. They will then transport more nutrient-carrying blood to the cochlea, and the transmission of sound waves will be greatly improved. This is the natural way to help protect against hearing loss and to restore healthy hearing.

A TWO-MINUTE EAR EXERCISE FOR
GREATER HEARING POWER

Loosen the congestion and accumulation of ear wax with a simple two-minute ear exercise that you can perform just about anywhere and any time.

Take your ear lobe between two of your fingers. Pull down *very gently*. Repeat this procedure up to fifteen times with each ear lobe. At the same time, make vigorous chewing motions as if you were chewing on something very hard.

Benefit: The rhythmic ear lobe pulling and chewing motion will help loosen the accumulation of decayed cells, wastes, impurities, and pollutants that have lodged in the crevices of your hearing organs. By loosening them through this two-minute exercise, you will help cleanse them of wastes.

HOW TO IMPROVE HEARING BY CONTROLLING NOISE POLLUTION

Noise pollution can create stress, which can elevate your blood pressure, constrict your arteries, and impede the flow of oxygen-carrying blood to your hearing organs. Prolonged exposure to noise pollution can produce involuntary responses by your audio-vascular systems and hearing organs and can create "shocks" that reduce hearing ability.

Hearing Loss Is Penalty for Noise Pollution. When otologists (ear specialists) measure noise levels and relate them to hearing loss, they note that regular exposure to noise at intensities of 85 decibels and frequencies greater than 3,000 cycles per second (those frequencies below 3,000 cycles per second are the most important for understanding speech) may result in serious hearing loss. Noise pollution may produce a permanent hearing loss due to weakening and destruction of certain inner ear structures. In particular, the microscopically small hairs in the inner ear that are responsible for conducting sounds to hearing nerves may be so damaged that eventual hearing loss occurs. So guard against noise pollution.

Basic steps to control noise pollution include:

1. Put carpets on the upper floors of your house to deaden the noise of footsteps.

2. Use heavy drapes in front of windows or outside walls to absorb noise from the outside and reduce the reverberation of sound within the room.

3. Use upholstered furniture and acoustical ceilings to minimize noise.

4. Seal windows to keep down outside noise.

5. Silence noisy plumbing by inserting neoprene or cork where pipes connect with other solid structures.

6. Replace loose or worn faucet washers to eliminate whistling or chattering noises.

7. Lower the setting on your heater thermostat to eliminate noises caused by very hot water.

8. Oil and repair mechanisms around the house so they are not so noisy. These include: ventilating fan over your stove, dishwasher, washing machine, garbage disposal unit, blender, any electrical or spring-driven mechanism, and vacuum cleaner.

9. Radios and televisions should be kept at a comfortable sound level so that they are easy on your ears and not abusive.

10. Recognize noisy areas in and around your home and working areas and try to avoid them or keep exposure to them to a bare minimum.

Noise Levels That Are Uncomfortable

The chart on page 103 tells you which noise levels are comfortable and which are uncomfortable. The chart shows you some noise levels to which you are exposed as well as the typical response to each level. "DBA" stands for "decibel" on the A scale, the unit used for measuring sound. Noise doubles approximately every 10 DBA. 90 DBA is twice as loud as 80 DBA. A reading of 80 DBA or over means the noise level is dangerous to your hearing and should be avoided as much as possible.

HOME REMEDIES TO HEAL AND REVITALIZE YOUR HEARING ORGANS

Revitalize your hearing organs with these home remedies for routine problems:

Earache. Susan Y. avoided chemical eardrops for her earaches because they left her skin red and itchy and often made her feel dizzy. She tried this easy, natural home remedy, recommended by a herbal pharmacist, to soothe her earache: Warm several drops of ordinary olive oil in a dry spoon above a match or candle. Test on the underside of your wrist to see if it's comfortable. Lie down with your bad ear up. Pour the comfortably warm olive oil into the ear. You will feel a soothing emollient action that eases the throbbing ache. Susan Y. found that repeated use of this home remedy offered a more permanent healing of the earache than chemical eardrops did.

Earwax. Combine one teaspoon of warm water with five drops of slightly warmed vegetable oil. Lie on your right side. Pour one-half of this solution into your left ear. Let it soak for about 60 seconds. Now place a clean cloth on the ear. Turn on your left side so that the excess solution is absorbed by the cloth. Pour the rest of this solution in your right ear. Let it soak about 60 seconds. Put clean cloth to your right ear to absorb the excess solution, and then sit up. The wax should be considerably softened. Remove gently with some soft

Effects of Noise Pollution on Your Hearing Organs

Source	Noise Level DBA		Effect on Speech	HEARING IMPAIRMENT
Power drill	140 130			Acute pain
Jet take-off (200 feet)	120			
Auto horn (3 feet)	110	Hearing damage at 1/2 hour per day		
Typical subway noise	100	Hearing damage at 2 hours per day	Shouting in ear	Discomfort
Heavy truck (25 feet)	90	Hearing damage at 8 hours per day	Shouting at 2 feet	Very annoying
Heavy traffic (rush hour)	85		Very loud conversa- tion at 2 feet	
Alarm Clock (3 feet)	80			
Vacuum Cleaner (10 feet)	70	Telephone use dif- ficult; noisy	Loud conversation at 2 feet	Annoyance threshold
Average home	50	Quiet	Normal conversation at 12 feet	Sleep interference
Whisper	30	Very quiet		
Breathing	10	Threshold of hearing		

cotton. You may have to repeat this procedure several times until stubborn wax is loosened and ready for removal.

Ear Pain. Make a poultice of chopped or grated raw onion and apply to the ear canal. Leave it on for up to 30 minutes. Ingredients in the onion tend to "draw away" the feeling of pain and give relief.

Ear Discomfort. If you feel discomfort in your ears in the form of a strain or pain, make a poultice out of chopped garlic and place this on the nape of your neck. Leave it on as long as is comfortably possible. Volatile oils in the garlic seep through the pores, warm the back of the neck (between your ears), and appear to relieve any discomfort.

Meniere's Disease. This is a generalized name given to problems such as repeated attacks of dizziness, nausea, ringing in the ears, and progressive deafness. This condition often occurs when the adrenal glands are exhausted. So much salt is lost that excessive fluid passes into the tissues at some focal point. Bacterial toxins may wash onto the auditory nerve and into the interior of the ear. The little bony structures suppurate (discharge pus), which indicates that nature wants corrections to be made. The body needs to be fortified with B vitamins, which can be found in whole grains, brewer's yeast, liver, nuts, wheat germ, bran, brown rice, soybeans, and whole grain cereals. These nutrients will convert sugars and starches into energy and thereby prevent their being stored in the bloodstream. They also help maintain better water balance in the system. They soothe the auditory nerves and help keep the ear organs clean.

Foreign Substance in Ear. An item such as an insect, a bean, or other debris that has gone into the ear can be removed by this simple method. Heat a little bit of oil in some water. When comfortably warm, put the solution into your ear so that the object can float out—it will usually do so.

Ringing in the Ears. Apply a heating pad to your feet and hands for as long as is comfortably possible. This will get to the *cause* of the ringing. Ringing is caused by pressure in the arterioles in the ears. There is pressure on the auditory nerve, which transports messages from the ear drum to the brain. A heating pad draws blood away from the parts of the body that are excessively congested. This redistribution improves circulation, relieves the pressure, and eases the ringing.

Ear Boils. Make a warm solution of water and a little salt. Use this solution as an ear wash. The salt helps destroy infectious bacteria and facilitate healing of boils and skin rashes.

BASIC CARE OF YOUR HEARING ORGANS

Keep things out of your ear canal. The old saying, "Never stick anything smaller than your elbow in your ear," is a wise one. If cotton is put in your ear, fibers may become imbedded in the ear wax and start the formation of a plug. Tiny splinters from match sticks may do the same thing. Above all, keep hard instruments away from your ear. They may scratch the lining of the ear and start an abscess, or they may force the wax against the ear drum.

Ordinary soap-and-water cleanliness for the outside of the ear is important to keep ear canals from being blocked. When you swim, dive, or bathe, keep water out of your nose, throat, and ear canal as much as possible. Wear a bathing cap with doctor-approved ear plugs when you swim.

If your face is under water, expel air slowly and continuously through your nose. If your face is above water, breathe in through your mouth. Practice in this is more important than learning a fancy stroke.

After swimming, or if you have a head cold, blow your nose gently, being sure that both nostrils are not closed at the same time. This helps keep wastes out of your eustachian tubes.

Avoid exposing your ears (and the rest of your body) to extreme temperature changes. If you are going from the warm indoors to the cold outdoors, wear ear muffs or cover your ears with your gloved hands. As your body adjusts to the temperature change, so will your ears.

Be rewarded with good hearing when you keep your ear organs in a condition of good health and revitalization with natural home programs.

IN A NUTSHELL

1. A physician used a three-step food program to restore his "lost" hearing.
2. After following the physician's three-step food program for only 21 days, a man enjoyed hearing restoration. Dizziness and ear ringing ended.
3. Two vitamins cured people of hearing loss, and nausea, ear ringing, and vertigo also vanished.

4. A high-vitamin, salt-free program improved hearing in many patients.

5. To hear better, try some of the easy exercises in this chapter. They only take a few moments.

6. Phyllis X. used a high-plant-food program to help restore hearing.

7. Boost the health of your ears with an easy, two-minute exercise.

8. Guard against noise pollution for greater ear health.

9. Susan Y. used a natural ear drop to ease her earache.

10. Soothe ear distress with easy-to-follow home remedies.

A Detoxifying Program
To Heal, Revitalize, and Rejuvenate Your Liver

8

Your liver is the sieve of your body. A clean and healthy liver will filter toxic elements from your system, release bile, which your body uses to metabolize food and help transform elements into digestible nutrients, and act as a storage site for important substances. As your body's sieve, your liver is a very important organ in relation to your metabolism and health. It is also the largest glandular organ in your body, and it may well be the most vital in helping to protect you against aging and illness.

Location of Your Liver. Weighing from three to four pounds, the liver is located on the right side of your abdomen, a little above your waistline. It is part of the digestive system. It can frequently be felt beneath the ribs.

Liver Is Part of Digestive Organ Network. Your liver is part of your basic digestive organ network. Channels from your liver join with a channel from your gallbladder (which is situated in a slight depression on the underside of the liver) to form a common channel that empties into the duodenum, a portion of the digestive system. Your liver is part of a network of organs that work together to filter and metabolize substances and maintain body health.

Your liver is an efficient sieve that filters out toxic wastes, and it must be kept in good health in order to function satisfactorily.

SIX LIVER-DETOXIFYING PROGRAMS FOR HEALING AND REVITALIZATION

To heal and revitalize your entire body, begin with your liver. Detoxify your body's sieve, and it will keep your digestive system clean and healthy. Here is a basic six-step program aimed at detoxifying your liver and building better health through healing and revitalization of your entire body.

1. Improving Clean Bile Flow

Organ Function: Each day, the liver manufactures about one pint of bile, which it releases to digest foods, especially fats, and metabolize them into a form that can be used to cushion your body and provide vitamins, minerals and proteins to all parts of your body. Bile needs to be clean in order to act as an efficient fat solvent.

Healing and Revitalization Program: John Mc D. had a problem with "bile backup." Whenever he ate his favorite foods—steaks, chops, and stews—he felt a burning sensation "wash" right up his throat. He felt painful rumbles in his stomach. If he lay down after a meal, the burning sensation was worse. He felt bloated. He looked sallow. John needed to make an adjustment in his food program. His physician outlined a simple healing and revitalization plan in which he *began* and *ended* each meat meal with *fresh, raw fruit.* John Mc D. began this plan immediately. The vitamins, minerals, and enzymes from the fruit were taken up by his liver and were used to clean the liver so that the bile flow was free of the sediment and fatty molecules deposited by the meats that John Mc D. loved. The liver took these nutrients and used them as a fat solvent so that the bile was "lighter" and less corrosive. The liver also used the nutrients from the fruits to improve its filtering powers. Now it could destroy some of the body's toxic wastes, changing them into waste products for elimination through the kidneys. The fruit nourished his liver and improved its ability to digest fats and direct the flow of bile so that it flowed into the digestive system instead of into the food gullet. John Mc D. could enjoy his delicious meats in all forms without any painful stomach rumbles or bloating. He no longer looked sallow. To further facilitate bile flow, he didn't lie down for at least one hour after eating. He would either sit or walk. This upright position helped his regenerated liver siphon bile into the proper ducts and in the proper downward direction. John Mc D. felt like a brand-new man, thanks to his clean bile program of raw fruit *before* and *after* each meat meal!

2. Improving Storage Power of Liver

Organ Function: One of the functions of the liver is to store food supplies for future use by your body. Digested sugars and starches are transformed into glycogen and stored in cells of the liver until they are needed by the body for energy. When your body signals a call for dextrose to give you vitality, your liver acts upon the demand. It converts the stored up glycogen into dextrose, an important blood sugar. Then your liver transports this dextrose to your tissues and muscles to give them the spark of youthful vitality.

Healing and Revitalization Program: Betty Z. looked wan, wasted, and haggard. Deep lines in her pale face made her look as exhausted as she felt. As a switchboard operator for a large firm, she needed to be alert to make instant connections and write down messages. But Betty Z. could not think quickly enough. She had to ask callers to repeat their names. She garbled up messages. By midday she felt as if she had gone through an entire day's work. Betty Z. was aware that something was wrong with her system. The company doctor told her that her clogged liver needed to be cleansed and supplied with energy-producing glycogen. Betty Z. healed and revitalized her "sluggish" liver with this tasty program: She drank four to six glasses of fruit juice throughout the day. The healing and revitalizing benefit of the fruit juice is its vitamins, minerals, and enzymes that can be rapidly assimilated by the digestive system. High energy fruits include oranges, grapefruits, tangerines, berries, peaches, plums, grapes. You can drink them separately or mix them.

Betty Z. discovered that the fresh juices acted as powerhouses of vitality. They almost "burst" with energy in her system. Her digestive system took the nutrients and sent them to her liver, which they cleansed of accumulated wastes. The liver took the natural carbohydrates of the juices, transformed them into glycogen, and stored them. Now, whenever Betty Z. needed energy, her liver released glycogen and gave her the vitality she required. She became a top-speed switchboard operator who rarely, if ever, made mistakes. She looked radiantly youthful, too, thanks to a healthy, glycogen-enriched liver.

3. Improving Iron-Storing Powers of Liver

Organ Function: Cells of the liver store iron, a mineral that enriches the bloodstream and guards against anemia. The liver slowly releases stored iron into the bloodstream, where it is used to form hemoglobin, the red coloring matter that carries oxygen from the lungs to all body cells. A clogged liver will be unable to store and release blood-building iron efficiently.

Healing and Revitalization Program: Troubled with cold hands, cold feet, a sickroom pallor, and constant chill even in the warm indoors, Edward De B. was miserable. He always had serious reactions to iron supplements, but he knew he had to "warm" up his body with iron. So he followed a tasty healing and revitalization program proposed by a nutritionist that worked to cleanse and detoxify his liver and boost its iron storing powers. Edward De B. mixed two tablespoons of *desiccated liver* with a glass of tomato juice. He drank this natural liver tonic twice daily. He also ate broiled or baked beef, chicken, or calf liver at least three times per week. With each broiled or baked liver dish, he ate a helping of *raw, fibrous vegetables,* such as carrots, radishes, celery, parsnips, and green peppers. They had to be raw, but for variety they could be shredded, diced, or chopped. This combination of foods had a unique liver-detoxifying and iron-building effect on Edward De B.

The desiccated liver and tomato juice tonic gave his liver a supply of iron that could be used for storage and distribution. The tomato juice provided a liquid medium by which the iron could "swim" to the liver for storage.

The combination of cooked liver and raw, fibrous vegetable provided two liver revitalization benefits. The cooked liver provided a powerhouse of important protein and iron for assimilation. The raw, fibrous vegetables acted as "liver scrubbers" in that the fibers of the vegetables cleared away debris and wastes and made the liver a healthy iron-storing and iron-distributing organ.

Edward De B. soon discovered that his limbs were warm, his face glowed with youthful health, and he was alert and cheerful. He felt like a man half his age. He regularly enjoys the desiccated liver and tomato juice tonic and the cooked liver and raw, fibrous vegetables.

Desiccated liver is dried, powdered beef liver, with the fat and connective tissue removed. It is a powerhouse of iron, protein, vitamins, and minerals. It is available at many pharmacies and at all health stores. A powdered or granular form is best since it can be stirred into tomato juice easily for swift assimilation.

4. Improving Poison-Filtering Powers of Liver

Organ Function: Pollution and chemicals in foods and beverages (including many drinking waters) carry metallic compounds that may impair the health of the liver. These poisons tend to accumulate in the liver and impair its filtering powers.

Healing and Revitalizing Program: Neutralize the corrosive effects of the poisons with a more healthful food program. Select fresh foods as often as possible. Avoid processed or chemicalized foods. If the water in your area has many contaminants, consider using bottled spring water for drinking and making beverages. Go on a raw juice fast frequently to wash your liver. Without the responsibility of metabolizing other foods, your liver can focus full attention upon assimilating the nutrients from fresh, raw fruit and vegetable juices. The vitamins, minerals, and enzymes in the juices help clean the tubules, ducts, filters, cells, and tissues of the liver. They help neutralize the corrosive effect of poisons from air and food pollution and also help sweep the poisons from your liver. A raw juice fast for one or two days will help clean your liver and boost its filtering powers so that it can keep you healthy and full of vitality.

5. Improving Digestive Powers of Liver

Organ Function: A healthy liver will be able to digest proteins efficiently, splitting them into amino acids which can be used by your body as building blocks of health and revitalization. A healthy liver assists in the manufacture of red blood cells, the creation of fibrinogen, which helps in blood clotting, and the storing of iron and copper. These processes help you resist infection, keep warm, and heal wounds and scratches by giving you enriched blood. Any impairment in the digestive powers of the liver will cause a reduction in these and many other health-building functions.

Healing and Revitalization Program: Do not abuse the digestive powers of your liver with harsh foods. Avoid the caffeine in coffee, cola drinks, and commercial teas. Avoid harsh, chemicalized seasonings, such as salt, pepper, ketchup, white vinegar, and mustard, and avoid foods made with these substances. Avoid the use of these seasonings in cooking and at the table. Use healthful items, such as Postum, herbal teas, and fruit and vegetable juices. Use healthful herbs and spices as seasonings. Almost all supermarkets carry these items. They are also available in nearly all health stores. Avoid alcohol and tobacco since these send burning poisons to the liver, which has to struggle harder to neutralize them. In the process, a poisonous residue is left clinging to the tubules and ducts, impairing their digestive powers. When you boost the health of your liver by avoiding harsh beverages and seasonings, you improve its protein absorbing mechanism and help your liver regenerate and to repair, revitalize, heal, and rejuvenate just about every part of your body. Be good to your liver, and it will reward you with better health.

6. Improving Health-Generating Powers of Liver

Organ Function: Your liver is full of health-generating powers if it is free of contamination and waste. Biliousness is a symptom of too much waste and unutilized food. Your liver cannot boost your health and symptoms of this problem include malaise, headache, fatigue, poor appetite, and weakness. When the liver has too many wastes, the liver cells producing digestive fluids become inflamed and congested. They tend to release too much of fluids such as bile. A healthy liver produces a beneficial and balanced supply of digestive liquids.

Healing and Revitalization Program: Begin each and every meal with a *subacid* fruit or juice. Acidic fruits include oranges, grapefruits, tangerines, lemons, limes, berries, grapes, nectarines, peaches, pears, pomegranates, sour apples, and cranberries. Use lemons and limes in moderation since they are potent. Mix them with other juices. *Tart subacid fruits* are quickly and easily digested. The liver need not drain these fruits of their elements. Instead, the liver will take some of the carbohydrates (they are minimal in subacid fruits and juices) and use the stronger elements for scrubbing away contamination. Furthermore, the liver will use the elements extracted from subacid fruits and juices to help normalize the flow of bile, which will neutralize toxic wastes accumulated in the liver cells. Subacid fruits and juices also clean the sensitive inner membrane of the intestines. They help create a better balance among the different digestive processes. They also break down any accumulations of wastes in the biliary tracts or channels that lead to the gallbladder and intestines. Heal and revitalize your liver with subacid fruits and juices. Use them at the start of your meal, and at the end if you want, so that your liver can cope with ingested food and regenerate at the same time. This is the easy way to heal and revitalize this important organ.

FOLK HEALERS FOR IMPROVED LIVER FUNCTION

Throughout the world, folklorists have recognized natural healers to improve the function of the liver. Here are some of these folk healers:

- *Beet and Celery Juice.* Mix one part beet juice with four parts celery juice. Drink several glasses of this mixture throughout the day.

- *Three-Way Juice.* Combine equal amounts of beet juice, celery juice, and carrot juice. Flavor this mixture with a bit of lemon juice if you'd like. Drink one glass of the mixture in the morning and another at night. Folklorists say that this Three-Way Juice works overnight to stimulate and detoxify the liver.

- *Herbal Tea.* In particular, folklorists recommend drinking an herb tea of dandelion and hops. Goldenseal is another favorite liver-cleansing tea. Folklorists suggest that you take no beverages other than herb teas for several days and eat healthful foods for effective liver-cleansing.

- *Lettuce Brew.* Chop up a small head of lettuce. Simmer the lettuce in just enough water to cover it. Then strain the lettuce and sip small amounts of the liquid throughout the day.

- *Raw Juice Fast.* For potent liver-cleansing, go on a raw juice fast for two days. Drink different fruit and vegetable juices and, if you'd like, herbal teas. A raw juice fast enables your liver to recuperate by bathing, washing, and scrubbing it in nutrient-rich juices without burdening it with nutrients from solid foods.

- *Laugh Tonic:* Enjoy a good, liver-healthy laugh. Folklorists say that a good laugh exercises the liver. It also exercises the diaphragm and the lungs and helps improve health in the entire body.

HEALING JAUNDICE WITH NATURAL METHODS

Jaundice is a symptom of a malfunctioning liver. It consists of a yellowing of the skin, the whites of the eyes, and even the mucous membranes. The cause of jaundice is an excess of bile pigment in the bloodstream. A healthy liver should dispose of wastes by converting them into urea, which is carried by the blood to the kidneys for elimination.

To correct jaundice, three things must be accomplished:

1. Any excess of bile pigment in the bloodstream must be liquefied and removed.

2. The liver cells must be made strong enough to remove excess bile pigment.

3. The bile ducts must be cleansed of obstructions so that bile can flow more freely without any sediment backup.

To heal and overcome jaundice, begin by correcting any liver disorders.

Food Program That Eliminated Jaundice. Marie G. would frequently fall victim to yellowing jaundice. She looked as if she would waste away. Medications left her dizzy. The longer she neglected the recurring jaundice, the worse it became. She was able to eliminate jaundice by going to the *cause* of the problem; namely, cleansing the liver so that it could act as a detoxifying organ and maintain a clean and balanced bile flow. A health spa physician prepared a simple healing program. Here is the program Marie G. followed that helped her recover and bounce back from jaundice:

High Protein Foods: Increase your intake of protein foods, especially fish, skim milk dairy products, peas, beans, nuts, whole grains, and some lean meat. *Healing Benefit:* The liver metabolizes the protein and uses the amino acids to help alert the digestive system to cleanse the bile ducts of obstructions. Amino acids become components of the liver cells enabling them to filter out impurities and normalize bile levels.

Fresh Juices Daily: Vegetable juices made from carrots, celery, tomatoes, lettuce, and cabbage are prime sources of enzymes and minerals needed to break down the accumulations of bile pigment in the bloodstream. *Healing Benefit:* Your liver can wash these wastes out through the juice-cleansed bile ducts. Fruit juices are also good sources of the vitamins that are needed to nourish the cells of the liver and revitalize them to make them more efficient.

Heat-Hydro Healer: It is very soothing to place warm, wet compresses on the liver and leave them to cool. *Healing Benefit:* The warmth opens your pores and lets the moisture enter to moisturize the parched segments of the liver and promote better cleansing of accumulated bile sediments. Use warm, wet compresses throughout the day.

Maintain Regularity: At breakfast time, have one or two glasses of prune or fig juice or a combination of two. You may also have a plate of pitted prunes as an item on your breakfast menu. Breakfast should also include whole grain cereal with bran and assorted seasonal, raw fruits. *Healing Benefit:* Regularity—freedom from constipation—means the body is being rid of accumulated wastes and toxic debris. Prunes, figs, and other fruits, and their juices, have a natural laxative effect on the bowels and intestines and help promote mobility. When jaundice is traced to obstruction, the intestines are "clogged" or "backed up." This obstruction can cause related organ difficulties because the kidneys and the gallbladder may also become clogged. Regularity helps ease liver problems and also eases jaundice.

Restrict Fried and Fatty Foods in All Forms: Fried and fatty foods are unhealthy for the liver and can contribute to jaundice and other disorders of the liver. When you are eating at home, bake, boil, broil, or steam your foods, but do not fry or add fatty grease to foods. *Healing Benefit:* When foods are fried or are fatty, fat globules are introduced to the system which tend to adhere to the ducts of the liver. Fatty globules are not easily dispersed. Cooking has coated the foods with a glue-like fatty coat that is difficult for the liver to remove. Clumps of fat break off from the coating and become lodged in the tubules and ducts of the liver and cause improper bile flow, which leads to jaundice. Avoid any foods that have been fried or are coated with fat. If you are eating out, ask the chef about his food preparation. If you are in doubt, stick to broiled or baked foods or stews and soups with a low-fat content.

The preceding five-step jaundice-easing program helps boost the power of your liver so that it can act as a free-flowing sieve—sparkling, clean, and vital, with youthful health.

A SWISS FOOD PROGRAM FOR HEALING OF LIVER UNREST

The Swiss believe that a three-day food program can heal and revitalize the liver and soothe liver unrest. Swiss nature healers prescribe this three-day food program:

Morning: One glass of carrot juice, one slice of whole grain bread or toast with a dab of oil, and some wheat germ in skim milk.

Noontime: Vegetable soup, brown rice or potatoes steamed in their jackets, and a raw carrot salad with bitter-tasting vegetables such as endive or chicory.

Evening: Oat, barley or brown rice soup with some chopped vegetables and a raw salad seasoned with lemon juice or yogurt.

For Variety: Tomato juice, whole grain sandwiches with nut butters, a cereal coffee (Postum) with a little skim milk, or salad of diced garlic, tomatoes, lettuce leaves, and a sprinkle of onion powder.

Avoid any coffee that contains caffeine, commercial teas, and cola drinks. To quench your thirst, try salt-free broth or bouillon.

Swiss healers say that the liver can regenerate itself within three days if this natural program is followed.

HOW OILS CAN LUBRICATE YOUR LIVER DUCTS

Free-flowing vegetable oils are prime sources of polyunsaturated fatty acids, which can help liquefy accumulated deposits and wash them out of your liver.

Improve Efficiency of Liver. Oils help promote efficiency of the liver. A lubricated liver is better able to store glucose in the form of glycogen and then release it as glucose to meet your energy needs. Specifically, vegetable oils moisturize the ducts. Oil prompts the liver to take *bilirubin,* an iron-free product of the breakdown of hemoglobin, and convert it to a form in which it can be discharged into the bile. Oil lubricates the liver ducts so that *bilirubin* can be removed from the blood and excreted into the bile. Without a sufficient intake of oil, or if the liver ducts are permitted to become coated with waste matter and fatty deposits, the *bilirubin* accumulates in the blood, pervades the tissue fluid, and causes a yellowing of the skin and the whites of the eyes because the flow of bile in the liver and outside it is obstructed. Some *bilirubin* is absorbed back into the bloodstream. With the help of oils in the daily diet, the liver ducts are washed free of obstructions. The *bilirubin* can be removed through the waste channels. Well-oiled liver ducts can create this healthy condition within the body's largest organ.

Oil for Salads, for Tonics, for Cooking. Use free-flowing vegetable oils as part of your salad dressing. You can also add two tablespoons of oil to any vegetable juice, stir the mixture vigorously (squeeze in a bit of lemon or lime juice for an added tang), and drink one glass of it daily. For any cooking that requires fat or grease, use free-flowing, golden oils from a vegetable source. Increase your intake of polyunsaturated oils, *available at almost any food store,* and improve the health of your liver.

ONE-DAY LIVER-DETOXIFYING PROGRAM

Because your liver is also a storage site, you should detoxify it regularly to keep your organs working efficiently. You may follow the same easy program used by Arthur O' L., a salesman, who had been looking wan and wasted, could not easily digest fat, and had recurring colds and allergies. He wanted to treat the *cause* of his problem rather than just the symptoms. So this busy salesman took the time to follow this simple one-day liver-detoxifying program, based on his readings in health publications:

Breakfast: High-protein, whole grain cereal (such as buckwheat, millet, bran, whole wheat, and wheat germ) in skim milk with iron-rich raisins and sun-dried apricots. Some fresh fruit. Yogurt with wheat germ and bran. Assorted seeds and nuts.

Luncheon: Broiled fish prepared with oils. Raw vegetable salad with oil, lemon juice, and vinegar. Whole grain rolls. Gelatin with cottage cheese topping. Herbal tea or caffeine-free coffee.

Dinner: Liver and onions broiled in oil. Waldorf or other salad with oil, lemon juice, and vinegar dressing. Whole grain bread. Vegetable broth. Herbal tea or caffeine-free coffee.

Liver-Cleansing Beverage: Three times daily, Arthur O' L. had a glass of vegetable juice with two tablespoons of vegetable oil. This *Liver-Cleansing Beverage* is high in enzymes, which propel the oil through the digestive system and help energize its polyunsaturates so that they can scrub the clogged ducts. Then the enzymes boost the action of the oil so that it can help push the *bilirubin* into the bile and wash it out of the body.

Natural Foods and Healthy Spices. Arthur O' L. restricted his intake of artificial and processed foods because they are full of liver-burning chemicals and additives. Instead, he ate only fresh foods. He avoided the use of any corrosive seasonings, such as salt in any form, sugar, pepper, white vinegar, mustard, ketchup, and relish. He used natural herbs and spices for flavoring and helped soothe his liver so that it could function efficiently.

Color Restored, Energy Boosted and Skin Made Youthful. In one day, his color was restored, he felt a surge of youthful energy, and his skin looked as young as he felt. Arthur O' L. felt his digestion improve, and he no longer suffered from his allergies. To help boost the efficiency of his liver, Arthur O' L. eliminated irritants from his regular diet. Soon, he recovered from his liver distress, and he had the energy and vitality of a young man.

Your liver is a sieve that must be kept healthy and clean so that it can work efficiently to cleanse your body of impurities. Detoxify your liver, and all of your other organs will benefit.

HIGHLIGHTS

1. Heal and revitalize your liver with a basic six-step program.

2. John Mc D. improved his bile flow and ended "bile backup" with an easy fruit program.

3. Betty Z. improved the storage power of her liver and recovered from premature aging. She boosted her vitality through a tasty program.

4. Edward De B. warmed his cold body through a special beverage and vegetable program.

5. Heal and revitalize your liver with tasty folk remedies.

6. Marie G. conquered jaundice with a simple liver-revitalizing program.

7. Ease liver unrest with a three-day Swiss food program.

8. Oils can lubricate your liver ducts for better health.

9. A One-Day Liver-Detoxifying Program cleanses the liver and boosts its power.

10. Arthur O' L. revitalized his liver with a simple program and a Liver-Cleansing Beverage.

How to Cleanse Your Kidneys
For Revitalized Circulation

9

Your kidneys are the master chemists of your body. They should be kept clean so that they can give you efficient circulation. Your kidneys are two of the most important life-giving organs of your body. If the kidneys fail, the body can't carry on. Healthy kidneys are essential to health and life. Let us take a closer look at these master chemists and see how to cleanse them for revitalized circulation and improved health.

Location and Description of Kidneys. Each person has two kidneys, one located on each side of the spine at the lowest level of the rib cage. In an adult, each kidney weighs about four ounces, is fist-sized, and is shaped like a kidney bean.

Each kidney contains about one million *nephrons.* A nephron consists of a collection of tiny blood vessels, called a *glomerulus,* and an attached tube, called a tubule. Through the nephrons pass fluids carrying nourishment and fluids carrying wastes to be removed.

You have about 140 miles of filters and tubes in both kidneys which perform the life-sustaining job of filtering body fluids and returning them to your bloodstream. Through your kidneys, this internal washing continues throughout your life.

During a 24-hour period, your kidneys filter some 200 quarts of liquids. About two quarts are sent to your bladder to be flushed out of your body. About 198 quarts are retained in your body.

HEALTHY KIDNEYS: SPACESHIP OF LIFE

A simple example taken from the flight of a spaceship will illustrate what healthy kidneys mean to your body and will clarify their basic importance to survival. A spaceship in flight has an apparatus that automatically controls temperature, humidity, and oxygen. No matter at what height the spaceship flies, the instruments adjust the atmosphere *within* the spaceship automatically so that the *internal environment* within the spaceship can support life. If the instruments were to fail, the environment within the ship would go bad and life within the spaceship would cease.

In the same way, healthy kidneys maintain a stable chemical composition of body fluids. They do this with the help of good nourishment and basic care. As long as your kidneys function efficiently, the internal environment can support life. If the kidneys fail, the body will falter, weaken, and die.

Kidneys Are Cleansing Organs. Your kidneys are cleansing organs, responsible for maintaining the delicate biological balance needed for all of the body organs to function efficiently. Healthy kidneys dispose of body wastes. They remove toxic substances from your bloodstream and retain substances that your body needs. That is why your kidneys can be called the "master chemists" of your body.

HOW TO PROTECT YOURSELF AGAINST KIDNEY STONES

What Are They? Kidney stones are gravel-like masses formed in the kidneys. Calcium salts, uric acid, and other substances crystallize out in the urinary tract and form masses that can block the drainage system of the kidneys. They range in size from a fine "gravel" to walnut-sized stones.

Corrective and Protective Methods: Very hot climates appear to predispose formation of stones. (The southeastern part of the United States is often called the "stone belt" because of the prevalence of this problem.) If you must live in a hot climate, arrange to have your home air-cooled. Try to work in an air-cooled environment, too.

Keep Your Body Active. An active body has less risk of forming kidney stones. People who sit for long periods of time (truck and bus drivers, pilots, office workers, or any other people with sedentary occupations or living habits) experience internal congestion and stagnation. This appears to predispose them toward formation of stones. Keep active. If you must sit, get up and walk around as often as possible. Take frequent walking breaks to stretch your legs, improve your circulation, boost the exchange of liquids, and promote better transportation of nutrients through the kidneys so that wastes will have less chance to accumulate.

A Kidney-Washing Program for Total Revitalization

Jeff K. came from a family with a history of kidney stones. He decided that he would not follow this pattern. He knew that he had to keep his kidneys cleansed so that accumulated wastes would not form kidney stones. So he followed this simple kidney-washing program, recommended by a nurse-dietician, that was tasty as it was revitalizing.

Apple Cider Vinegar and Water Mixture Three Times Daily. Jeff K. prepared an apple cider vinegar and water drink to take *before* each meal. Into a glass of ordinary fruit juice, he stirred three tablespoons of pure apple cider vinegar, which is available at most health stores and supermarkets. He added half a teaspoon of honey for flavoring and stirred the mixture vigorously. He drank one glass of this mixture *before* each meal. Jeff K. found that this simple program gave him a feeling of exhilaration, revitalized him, and protected him from the kidney stones that had plagued others in his family.

Benefit: Apple cider vinegar is a prime source of highly concentrated pectin and hemicellulose, as well as of fruit acids. These substances act as catalysts in that they are able to disperse and then distribute accumulated wastes that threaten to lodge within the kidneys. When apple cider vinegar, fruit juice, and a bit of honey are taken *before* a meal, the ingredients initiate a kidney-activation program. The ingredients help scrub away accumulated debris so that the kidneys are clean and can accommodate the nutrients ingested from the upcoming meal. Taken *before* a meal, this mixture alerts and activates the kidneys and stimulates a "scrubbing" of the nephrons so that debris is washed away. This is a natural way to protect yourself from kidney stones.

HOW TO COOL AND REFRESH INFLAMED KIDNEYS

Bright's disease, or nephritis, is a condition in which the kidneys become inflamed. There may be albumin (protein substance) in the urine as well as swelling (edema) of some body tissues. These symptoms indicate that the kidneys are weak in their filtering responsibilities and that the delicate glomerular membrane is fragile, which allows the escape of important protein. To cool, refresh, and rebuild the inflamed kidneys and prevent the risk of Bright's disease, follow this basic healing program:

1. *Eliminate Salt from Food Program.* Salt is a corrosive. It is filtered through the kidneys. The kidneys can handle only a small amount of salt, and when they are overburdened they must work harder and harder, which causes a breakdown. Eliminate salt from the table and in cooking. Select products without added salt. Use natural herbs and spices for flavoring. Salt is an acid food that is scorching to the delicate tubules of the kidneys and may cause kidney breakdown. It should be restricted from your food program.

2. *Drink Eight to Ten Glasses of Liquids Daily.* Throughout the day, drink large amounts of liquids as a means of helping to moisturize accumulated foodstuffs and thereby ease the burden of the kidneys as filtering agents. Drink fresh water, lots of fruit and vegetable juices, soup, herbal teas, and broths. You may also eat lots of succulent fruits and vegetables, which are high in liquid content. Many beverages and plant foods contain nutrients that nourish and rebuild the tubules and cells of the kidneys to strengthen them so that they can work more efficiently.

3. *Eliminate Caffeine From Your Menu.* Caffeine acts as an irritant to the kidneys and may be involved in destroying their delicate tissues. Avoid the caffeine in coffee, tea, chocolate, cocoa, soft drinks, and cola beverages. Replace these beverages with coffee substitutes such as Postum, herbal teas, fruit and vegetable juices, soups, and broths. These beverages are kind to your kidneys. They will soothe and rebuild the nephrons and tubules so that there is less risk of "leakage" and Bright's disease.

4. *Eliminate Tobacco and Alcohol.* These products contain chemicals that are harmful to kidneys. Nicotine and alcohol contain poisonous substances that act to burn and inflame the kidneys. These organs are forced to filter out these poisons, and in the process the delicate cells and tissues become broken, damaged, and destroyed. Some of the poisons are absorbed by the kidneys, and the threat of Bright's disease is great. Be kind to your kidneys and your health in general by eliminating tobacco and alcohol in any form.

5. *Avoid Temperature Extremes for Better Kidney Health.* Foods and beverages should be of a comfortable temperature, neither too hot nor too cold. Shocking your kidneys with overly hot items or

ice-cold items can cause internal damage and inflammation similar to that of Bright's disease, or nephritis. CAUTION: Do NOT follow hot food immediately with cold food. The constrast in temperature acts as a *shock* to your kidneys and may cause reduced function. It disturbs your body's thermoregulatory system, and your kidneys become scorched and then frozen in a matter of minutes. This seesawing in temperature is unhealthy. Foods and beverages should be comfortably hot or comfortably cool when consumed. Avoid extremes. Your kidneys will be thankful for this kindness.

A "P-C" PROGRAM THAT REVITALIZED "SLUGGISH" KIDNEYS

Amy O' N. was troubled with a "sluggish" kidney that she feared could result in the formation of stones or inflammation. She was worried about her "cloudy" urine. Sometimes she felt a burning sensation during voiding. She began to look worn out. Her skin started to sag. She developed rashes and skin infections that did not clear up easily. Amy O' N. was told by a specialist that she displayed symptoms like those of nephritis and that much protein was being lost from her body, causing tissue breakdown. She had to make a simple dietary adjustment that she called a "P-C" Program.

How the "P-C" Program Revitalized Sluggish Kidneys

Two food elements—protein and Vitamin C—formed the basis of Amy O' N.'s basic program. She planned for each of her meals to include as much of these elements as possible.

Protein is found in meat, fish, eggs, cheese, peas, beans, nuts, and seeds.

Vitamin C is found in citrus fruits, such as oranges, lemons, limes, tangerines, grapefruits, and tangelos, and in tomatoes, green peppers, and berries.

Protein and Vitamin C Lead to Kidney Revitalization. Amy O' N. built her daily menu around these two food elements. For breakfast she had a soft boiled egg with half a grapefruit, among other items. For lunch she had broiled fish with an assortment of seasonal fruits from the Vitamin C group. For dinner she had lean meat or a peas and beans and brown rice mixture with various Vitamin C fruits. She drank juices from the Vitamin C group frequently. It took eight days for Amy O' N. to discover the change. She no longer had cloudy urine. The burning sensation was gone. Her skin tightened up and became clear and youthful again. Soon her revitalized kidney restored her to youthful health. She follows her "P-C" Program that is kind to her kidneys and revitalizing to her entire body regularly!

Benefits of a "P-C" Program: When you emphasize and increase your intake of high-protein and high-Vitamin C foods daily, you help heal your kidneys. Inflammation in the kidneys involves the glomerular membrane and results in the escape of large amounts of protein from the bloodstream into the urine. As a result of this protein loss, large quantities of water accumulate in the body and body breakdown may begin. But this condition can be corrected with a *combination* of protein and Vitamin C. Your metabolism takes the protein and uses it to rebuild the glomerular membrane and replace the protein that is being lost in waste. At the same time, your metabolism is energized by Vitamin C to form *collagen,* which is a cement-like substance that heals, knits, and strengthens the tubules and membranes of the kidneys so that there is eventual correction of protein leakage. A "P-C" program emphasizes the importance of these substances so that they can heal and revitalize the kidneys and boost the health of your entire body!

A FIVE-MINUTE TEST FOR KIDNEY HEALTH IN YOUR OWN HOME

Normal urine is a clear amber color and is slightly acid. Passage of urine should be comfortable. If you void urine that is very dark and is irritating, it may be nature's warning signal that something is wrong with your kidneys. You can conduct a five-minute test of your urine in your own home that will tell you whether your kidneys are in need of revitalizing. To do so, you need to obtain some Nitrazine Paper, which is available at any pharmacy and many health stores for a very modest price. Here is an explanation of this test.

Acid-Alkaline Balance, or pH. The pH of a substance is a measure of acidity or alkalinity of the substance. It is expressed on a scale whose values run from 0 to 14, with 7 representing neutrality, 0 being highly acid, and 14 being highly alkaline.

A reading of pH 4.5 to 5.5 or 6 for urine is average.

How to Test Your Urine Acidity. Test your first and second morning voidings. Dip a strip of Nitrazine Paper into the urine, shake off excess fluid, and read the paper immediately, using the color chart that is part of the Nitrazine Paper package. This test will tell you, within a few moments, the degree of acidity or alkalinity of your urine.

- A reading of below 7.0 indicates an acid level.
- A reading of above 7.0 indicates an alkaline level.

Avoid Extremes. If your reading is very much below 7.0, you have too much acid in your urine. If your reading is very much above 7.0, you have too much alkali in your urine. A healthy *balance* is indicated by a reading of 4.5 to 5.5 or 6.

If your five-minute home test shows either extreme, it suggests that your kidneys are either too acid or too alkaline. You can be kind to your kidneys by balancing the pH levels with proper nutrition.

Foods That Raise Acid Levels: High-protein foods such as meat, fish, eggs, gelatin products, and such fruits as cranberries, plums, and prunes. Drinking cranberry juice is an excellent and tasty way to raise your acid level.

Foods That Raise Alkali Levels: All dairy products, including milk, buttermilk, cheese, and yogurt, and most vegetables and citrus fruits and their juices. Your metabolism will use acid citrus fruits to stimulate and produce an alkaline urine.

Take the five-minute test frequently and heed nature's signals to balance the acid-alkali levels of your system and wash your kidneys with soothing liquids.

COMMON AND UNCOMMON KIDNEY-REVITALIZING HOME REMEDIES

Energize and revitalize your kidneys (and entire body) with these home remedies:

Asparagus for Healing. This everyday vegetable contains *asparagine,* a natural catalyst that creates a strong kidney-washing effect. It also helps to counteract the effects of oxalic and uric acids (corrosives) in the kidneys. Eat asparagus regularly for its good taste and its kidney-cleansing effects.

Barley Water. Add two ounces of barley (the non-pearled or unpolished kind, available in health stores) to two quarts of boiling water. Let the liquid boil until it is reduced to one quart. When it is comfortably warm, drink a glass of it. Leave the rest of it in the refrigerator (in a covered glass container) until you are ready to use it. Then drink it at a comfortably cool (but not cold!) temperature.

It is a soothing mucilaginous beverage, and it moistens the kidneys, nourishing them with minerals and polyunsaturated fatty acids so that they can be revitalized for better health.

Citrus Juice Fast. For one day, try a Citrus Juice Fast. Take no other foods or juices. Citrus juices are prime sources of enzymes and Vitamin C. When they are sent pouring into your digestive system, the enzymes speedily take the Vitamin C and help dissolve toxic wastes and prevent formation of renal calculi (kidney stones). They also help to keep the urine free of these deposits. When citrus juices can bathe the kidneys without interference from other foods or juices, they can work with effective force in cleaning debris and revitalizing the tubules, cells, and tissues. Just one day on this tasty program will do much to heal and revitalize your kidneys.

Herb Tea for Kidney Healing. Health stores have a special herb tea available that helps heal kidneys. *Fenugreek tea* acts as a solvent to cleanse and remove accumulations of decayed cells and wastes. Fenugreek tea loosens hardened matter from within the kidney tubules and then cleans and soothes the membranes. A tasty beverage, especially with some lemon juice and honey, it should be enjoyed daily for kidney and body health.

Eliminate Oxalic Acid Foods. Oxalic acid causes the accumulation of calcium oxalate crystals, which can combine and form stones. Either reduce or eliminate foods that are very high in oxalic acid: spinach, cocoa, black tea, rhubarb, beet leaves, coffee, sweetbreads, thymus, spleen, and lungs. *Suggestion:* Drink lots of water between meals. Also, drink fresh fruit and vegetable juices. These help dissolve oxalate crystals that may build up from other everyday foods.

Parsley Tea. Folklore healers have frequently prescribed two or three glasses of parsley tea daily as a means of helping to heal and revitalize sluggish kidneys. To make parsley tea, boil one bunch of store-sized parsley in two pints of water for 15 minutes. Let the tea cool and then drink it. You can flavor it with lemon juice and honey. Nutrients in the parsley appear to stimulate the activity of the kidneys.

Always Keep Feet Warm. Have you ever suddenly plunged or stepped into a cold environment and had the urge to urinate? This may happen if you walk with warm feet on a cold floor, if you put warm feet in cold water, or if you are caught in a rain shower and get your feet wet. The bladder telegraphs signals to your kidneys, and the urge to void occurs. *Always keep your feet warm, and always avoid temperature shocks!* If you don't, the soles of your feet may cause the contraction of the blood vessels in the bladder, which creates a disturbance of the muscles involved in the kidneys and triggers a voiding urge. This sudden urge forces the kidneys into an activity they may not have to perform, thereby causing stress and tension. This weakens kidney health. So always be sure to keep your feet warm whether you are in bed, walking, sitting, or standing. *Never* allow your feet to be shocked in a cold environment.

HEALING YOUR KIDNEYS WITH
WATER THERAPY AT HOME

Activate your kidneys and improve their self-cleansing with water therapy at home. Water has a natural therapeutic effect. If cool, it stimulates the superficial nerve endings of the kidneys. If warm, it soothes and relaxes them.

You may take regular baths, which tend to comfort the entire body. You may also use some of these specific kidney-comforting water therapies:

Cool Water Pack. Soak a thick piece of cloth (long enough to reach around your abdomen and the small of your back) in comfortably cool water. Wrap it around your middle like a sash. Cover the cloth with a dry towel and leave it on for a few hours. Replace it with a newly soaked cloth when it dries. *Kidney-Healing Benefit:* The cool comfort gently contracts small skin blood vessels and helps to dilate or open the internal vessels to stimulate the kidneys into a brief contraction. It is an effortless "exercise" for sluggish kidneys.

Warm Water Pack. Soak a thick piece of cloth (long enough to reach around your abdomen and the small of your back) in hot water. Squeeze out the water. (Be careful not to burn your hands.) When it is comfortable to the touch, wrap it around your middle like a sash. Cover it with a dry towel. Leave it on until it is cool. Replace it with a new cloth. Continue this procedure for one hour. *Kidney-Healing Benefit:* The warmth of the water relaxes tense muscles and relieves congestion in the kidneys and related organs through a reflex response of the spinal nerves. Circulation is improved. The peripheral blood vessel balance is improved.

Contrast Baths. Plan to "exercise" your kidneys through the use of contrasting *comfortably* warm and *comfortably* cool baths. If possible, obtain a bath spray attachment (at houseware outlets) and direct the comfortably warm water to the small of your back for five minutes. Then change to a comfortably cool water spray to the same area. The temperature stimulates your kidneys, "wakes them up," increases metabolism, and helps promote excretion of infections and toxins. Try this Contrast Bath several times a week. First use five minutes of warm water, then five minutes of cool water, then five minutes of warm water, and then a final five minutes of cool water. Towel dry and feel exhilarated through revitalized kidneys.

Epsom Salt Bath. This old-fashioned but highly effective therapy was used by Oscar La B. when he experienced inflammation, sluggishness, and difficulties in voiding. Oscar La B. corrected these problems with this very easy Epsom Salt Bath. Run water temperature to about 100° F. Add two pounds of Epsom salts (also known as magnesium sulfate, available at pharmacies and many health stores) to the warm water. Now soak yourself for up to 20 minutes. You should be perspiring. Stand under tepid water and shower off the Epsom salts. Dry yourself. Cover yourself with warm blankets and do *not* go anywhere until you are fully dry. *Kidney-Healing Benefit:* A comfortably warm Epsom Salt Bath tends to stimulate the kidneys to boost elimination of uric and oxalic acids through the open skin pores. Blood alkalinity tends to improve. Toxins are washed out. You are internally cleansed. The "washed" kidneys now make you feel revitalized. You can help heal your kidneys (and body) with an Epsom Salt Bath several times a week. Make it part of your total body revitalization program.

Salt Glow. A time-tested folk healer, the Salt Glow seems to stimulate the action of the kidneys to throw off accumulated toxins and soothe the inflammation of Bright's disease. It's quite simple. Add water to ordinary table salt until it is of a paste-like consistency. Stand or sit in your tub and rub this salt paste over your entire body. Rub gently but firmly into the small of your back near your kidneys. Rub yourself until you feel yourself glowing. Then wash off the salt paste with a contrasting warm and cool shower or body spray.

Inhalation Therapy. Breathe new life into your kidneys with the use of pine-needle extract, peppermint oil, and spearmint oil. These are available at many health stores and herbal pharmacies. Add a small amount of any of these herbs to comfortably warm bath water. As you soak in the water, breathe deeply. The vapors of these woods and field herbs will soothe the lining of your air passages and respiratory organs and will also soothe your other vital organs. The kidneys appear to be benefited by herbal inhalation therapy. Herbal inhalation therapy is as fresh and invigorating as the woods and mountains. It stimulates the kidneys so that they function more healthfully.

Your kidneys benefit from water therapy that causes profuse and healthy perspiration. Profuse perspiration casts out accumulated toxins so that the kidneys can work healthfully to help you enjoy better living.

Water therapy helps to correct "stasis," or the formation of pools of waste in which bacteria can grow and multiply. By using simple and effective water therapy, you can help heal and revitalize your kidneys and help them to regulate normal voiding.

Your kidneys act with water to filter wastes out of the blood and return blood cells and proteins to the bloodstream. This job is made easier when you are kind to your kidneys and use wholesome methods to heal and revitalize them and the rest of your body.

SUMMARY

1. Protect yourself from kidney stones by working in an air-cooled environment, keeping yourself active, and drinking lots of liquids.
2. Jeff K. followed a simple Apple Cider Vinegar and Water Mixture program to guard against kidney stone development.
3. Cool and refresh inflamed kidneys and guard against Bright's disease, or nephritis, with a basic five-step program.
4. Amy O' N. followed a "P-C" Program to revitalize her sluggish kidneys. She cleared up her "cloudy" urine and ended the burning sensation during voiding.
5. Try the five-minute test for kidney health in your own home.
6. Heal and revitalize your kidneys with the various home remedies outlined in this chapter.
7. Heal your kidneys with a variety of different water therapies.
8. Oscar La B. cooled inflammation and eliminated voiding difficulties with a simple 20-minute Epsom Salt Bath.

How to Pamper Your Gallbladder
For Internal Rejuvenation

10

Be good to your gallbladder. Pamper it for improved fitness and internal rejuvenation. This organ works together with your liver to emulsify and digest fat. It also acts as a storage depot for bile, a substance that is needed for the digestion of fats. To pamper your gallbladder so that it will reward you with better fat metabolism, you must nourish it with certain foods and keep it free from accumulated debris.

Location of Gallbladder. The gallbladder is a pear-shaped pouch situated on the undersurface of the liver in the upper right part of the abdomen just below the diaphragm.

Function of Gallbladder. The gallbladder stores and concentrates liver-dispatched bile, a dark-colored fluid that helps in the digestion of fats. Between meals, when bile is not needed, it is stored in the gallbladder. When food is consumed, the tube from the gallbladder opens and bile flows into the intestine.

How Bile Metabolizes Food. Bile has no digestive enzymes. It helps in the digestion of food by attacking the large globules of fat and breaking them into small droplets that can be easily digested by fat-splitting enzymes in your system. Bile then works to remove layers of undigested fat on protein and carbohydrate foods in the intestine to enable enzymes to metabolize them and prepare them for use by the body. If there is not enough bile available, the protein and carbohydrate foods remain covered with the layers of undigested fat because enzymes cannot break down this fat alone. Therefore, the fat remains undigested, which prompts the growth of harmful bacteria and the formation of gallstones. Bile must be present in sufficient quantities. This is possible through correct nutrition.

BALANCED BILE SUPPLY PROTECTS AGAINST GALLSTONE FORMATION

A balanced supply of bile is the key to protection against gall-stone formation. Gallstones (*biliary calculi*) are formed when there is an accumulation or stagnation of bile in the gallbladder. If bile cannot flow freely from the gallbladder, it backs up. Faulty diet may result in an unbalance in the amounts of cholesterol and bile salts, and accumulation begins. Gallstones are almost pure cholesterol. They are deposited in the gallbaldder and form balls. They may be as tiny as pinheads or as large as golf balls. When the diet is too high in animal fats, overstimulation of the gallbladder occurs, which leads to an excess of bile. Not all of this bile can be accommodated by the body, and stones may form. To protect against this health risk, a balanced food program is important.

A DOCTOR'S DIET FOR GALLBLADDER RELIEF[1]

A physician has prepared a tasty food program that will help protect you from excess bile formation, ease painful contractions, and prevent stones.

Benefit of Low-Fat Diet. Since a high cholesterol and fat intake appears to initiate formation of gallstones, the following low-fat program may be beneficial. If bile does not flow properly into the intestines, fats may be poorly absorbed, which may cause indigestion. A low-fat diet is gentle because it spares the liver, which might otherwise be harmed by a backwash of bile from the gallbladder. Here is the doctor's food program that can pamper your gallbladder:

Foods Allowed

Soups: Vegetable, clear, without cream or fat.

Meats: Should be lean. Use lamb, beef, white meat of chicken and turkey, and any type of tender, well-cooked meat, except those listed in the Foods to Be Avoided section below. Also use fish.

Vegetables: These should be well cooked. But avoid beans, either baked or fried.

---

[1] *Parker Natural Health Bulletin,* Vol. 7, No. 1, January 3, 1977, West Nyack, New York 10994. Available by subscription.

Fruits: Oranges, lemons, grapefruit, apples, and any type of stewed fruits *without* the skins.

Salads: Any type of fruit salad without oil. Avoid raw vegetables.

Cereals and Cereal Products: Any type of cereal, wheat, barley, brown rice, and tapioca. If you are overweight, you should either omit these or use them sparingly, without sugar or cream. Bread should be used in moderation (or avoided if you are overweight). Graham, rye, or toasted white bread and hard rolls may be used. Bread must be stale.

Desserts: Junkets, ices, gelatin, and light puddings. Use sparingly, without cream sauces and with the white of an egg.

Foods to Be Avoided

Avoid all fat, greasy foods, soups, gravies, sauces, and so on. Cream and butter are to be used sparingly or not at all. All fatty meats and game should be avoided. Eggs may be used in moderation (about three per week). Sweetbreads, liver, and kidney should be avoided.

Avoid all fried foods, spiced foods, and foods prepared with or canned in oil. Avoid condiments, spices, pickles, and, in general, all coarse or rich, heavy dishes. Alcohol and salty foods should be avoided. If you are overweight, sugar and starch should be used in moderation.

Generally speaking, avoid overeating. It is soothing to your gallbladder to eat small meals with small snacks between meals. Avoid large meals. Water may be taken as desired.

THE FAT THAT FLATTERS YOUR GALLBLADDER

Joan R. suffered painful contractions whenever she ate some of her favorite foods. There were times when the pain ran right up to her shoulder blade. The recurring spasms made it difficult for Joan R. to eat even very lean cuts of her favorite meats. She was told by a local health clinic nutritionist that on her current program, in which she excluded almost all fat, she was actually harming her gallbladder. She was told that if she began each of her meals with a simple, everyday food, she could soothe her gallbladder so that is would be contented and pampered.

Olive Oil Soothes Gallbladder. Joan R. took three tablespoons of ordinary olive oil before each meal. She washed it down with tomato juice, when she found it too oily for her taste. She then followed a moderate low-fat program. Soon the painful contractions subsided. The pains and spasms went away. Now she can enjoy many of her favorite foods without any of the aftereffects, thanks to the olive oil.

Revitalizes Gallbladder and Balances Bile Flow. This simple, everyday food, olive oil, is a monounsaturated fat. It neither raises nor lowers cholesterol levels, but it does revitalize the gallbladder by helping it maintain a balanced bile flow. The bile assimilates the fat-soluble vitamins A, D, E, and K. Because olive oil is a mono-unsaturated fat, it is *gentle* to the gallbladder. It *balances* bile flow with virtually no contractions. Olive oil taken *before* a meal is especially beneficial since it prepares the gallbladder and prompts it to release bile to handle the oncoming fats with vigor and youthful effectiveness.

Just three tablespoons of olive oil, taken three times daily (preferably a half hour before mealtime), will do much to help improve the health of your gallbladder.

HOW PLANT FOODS AND JUICES HELP MELT AND DISSOLVE GALLSTONES

A victim of gallstones, Andrew MacM. suffered stomach upset with chemical medicines. He had painful rumblings whenever he ate some of his favorite foods. At times, he felt knife-like sensations that caused him to double over in agony. He felt as trapped as his gallstones! He was willing to follow any program that would offer relief and freedom from gallstones. So it was that he followed a physician-outlined, three-day, natural plant food program that so invigorated his gallbladder that he felt that his gallstones had been melted and dissolved. Andrew MacM. discovered "freedom from gallstones" with this program:

First Day: A variety of vegetable juices that were to be sipped slowly. At least five to six glasses of different vegetable juices throughout the day. Steamed seasonal vegetables with a bit of olive oil and some honey for a dressing. Three or four meals consisting of any combination of steamed vegetables. (Beans were not allowed.)

Second Day: Four to six glasses of fruit juices throughout the day. A variety of stewed fruits (without the skins) flavored with a bit of honey. Fresh, seasonal fruit, peeled, could also be eaten throughout the day. Three or four meals consisting of favorite stewed or fresh fruits.

Third Day: The *first half* of the day consisted of a raw fruit juice fast. No foods to be taken. No other beverages (except water). The *second half* of the day consisted of a raw vegetable juice fast. No other foods to be taken. No other beverages (except water).

Benefit of Three-Day Plant Food and Juice Fast: Ordinarily, gallstones are formed when bile becomes thickened due to too many fatty and indigestible foods. Bile normally flows rapidly through the ducts of the gallbladder. But when bile is thick, the flow is sluggish and the gallbladder does not completely empty. The remaining bile precipitates, causing stone formation. A *Three-Day Plant Food and Juice Fast* sends a shower of enzymes (from the raw plant foods and juices) to the gallbladder to *liquefy* thickened bile and help break up the hardened crystals and wash out the accumulated debris. This helps to loosen and dissolve hardened toxic wastes and pass them out of the body. During a fast, body organs are relieved of the obligation to metabolize animal fats. They can focus their full efforts and vigor upon the stored materials in the body. They turn inward and, with the enzymatic propulsion powers of plant foods, are able to "attack" the hardened crystals and dissolve them out of the body. It is the natural way to help discover freedom from gallstones.

HOW HERBAL REMEDIES HELP DISSOLVE GALLSTONES

A physician, R. Swinburne Clymer, M.D.,[2] says: "In many instances, it is possible to dissolve formed gallstones or to prevent their formation by proper medication." Dr. Clymer offers these two natural tonics as effective treatments for gallstones. The ingredients are available at most herbal pharmacies. The herbal pharmacies may be able to prepare these "natural prescriptions" for gallstone dissolving:

Natural Prescription #1

Tincture of Tetterwort (*Sanguinaria canadensis*) . . 5 to 10 drops

Tincture of Barberry (*Berberis vulgaris*) . . . . 3 to 5 drops

Tincture of Fringe Tree (*Chiolanthus virginica*) . . . 3 to 5 drops

Tincture of Bitter Root (*Apocynum
androsaemifolium*) . . . . 1 to 2 drops

---

[2]*Nature's Healing Agents* by R. Swinburne Clymer, M.D. Dorrance and Co., Philadelphia, Penna., 1963.

Take the mixture in water three times a day. It is best to take it 30 minutes after meals.

Natural Prescription #2

Tincture of Wormseed .... 8 to 10 drops

Tincture of Rheumatism Root (*Discores villosa*) .. 1 to 5 drops

Tincture of Mandrake (*Podophyllum peltatum*) ... 1 to 3 drops

Tincture of Fringe Tree (*Chiolanthus virginica*) ... 3 to 5 drops

Take the mixture in water three to four times a day.

EVERYDAY FOODS THAT HEAL AND REVITALIZE YOUR GALLBLADDER

A balanced diet that is high in essential nutrients will do much to help heal and revitalize your gallbladder and entire body. An abundance of vitamins, minerals, proteins, enzymes, natural carbohydrates, polyunsaturated fatty acids, and trace elements helps establish organ-harmony and balance. These nutrients build and rebuild components of your gallbladder and other organs and help improve health. Some foods have been singled out as especially helpful in healing and revitalizing the gallbladder. These are everyday foods that are tasty and are effective in improving the gallbladder. They are considered folklore health remedies, but they have been shown to be effective in organ healing. These foods are available everywhere for a modest cost.

ALFALFA. An unusually rich source of minerals because its roots dig down as much as 100 feet in the soil to absorb minerals from the earth. These minerals help nourish the tubules and tissues of the gallbladder.

ALMONDS. Just one pound offers well over a thousand milligrams of magnesium, which is needed by your gallbladder for the formation of cell-building proteins. Also, help activate enzymes to promote better metabolism of nutrients involved in gallbladder healing.

APRICOTS. An unusually rich source of iron and copper, which are needed by the gallbladder for better blood.

BEETS: Discard the greens because they are high in oxalic acid. Use the bulbous or root portions, which are rich in vitamins as A, B, and C and potassium, calcium, phosphorus, and sulfur. Beets appear to act as a cleanser of the gallbladder, loosening debris and helping to protect against formation of crystals.

BLACKBERRIES. A rich source of tannic acid, which enriches the bloodstream and acts as an astringent for the gallbladder. Has a good alkaline reaction to offset hyperacidity in this region.

BLUEBERRIES. A high mineral food that helps purify and fortify the bloodstream. Blueberries also contain *myrtillin,* a natural gallbladder food that reduces excess blood sugar and acts as a form of natural insulin for the neighboring pancreas. Soothes this area.

CELERY. High in minerals and vitamins and helps create natural roughage that sweeps out accumulated wastes around the gallbladder. Celery juice will also act as a natural diuretic to wash out the gallbladder.

CHERRIES. Especially beneficial because of their nutrients and citric and malic acids, which work to neutralize uric acid in the bloodstream and thereby prevent the "backwash" of burning noted in gallbladder unrest. Raw cherries or cherry juice may be enjoyed.

CITRUS FRUITS. The gallbladder will be healed by vitamins that are found in the white netting under the peel of citrus fruits. Try a squeeze of lime juice in comfortably warm water for a natural cleansing. A glass of grapefruit juice helps to scrub away accumulated grease and fats from the tubules of the gallbladder. It also helps to liquefy bile so that there is less risk of hardening.

CUCUMBERS. A prime source of *erepsin,* a protein-metabolizing enzyme that transforms nutrients into amino acids that heal and revitalize the gallbladder. Use regularly for salads. Do NOT use commercial pickles, which are treated with brine and acid. Select firm cucumbers. If the cucumbers are not organic, peel them before using.

DATES. A prime source of alkaline substances to offset acid buildup. Also contains minerals needed to nourish the gallbladder.

GRAPES. Eat regularly to offset any acid backwash in the gallbladder. They help wash out accumulated uric acid from the system. Eat grapes and enjoy grape juice for healing and revitalizing of your gallbladder.

LETTUCE. A good roughage food. It is alkaline and will soothe the burning of acid buildup. Promotes better elimination. Helps pamper your gallbladder and soothe it.

NUTS. Nuts are prime sources of vegetable protein and polyunsaturated fats, which are needed to nourish and heal the gallbladder. They are especially beneficial because they (and seeds) are free of uric acid.

PAPAYA. A juicy fruit. Its ingredients tend to cleanse, normalize, and detoxify the gallbladder.

PUMPKIN SEEDS. Especially beneficial in helping wash out debris from the bile solution to keep it free-flowing and clean. Eat pumpkin seeds raw, throughout the day. If you have a seed grinder, pulverize them and use them for baking.

SOYBEANS. Higher in protein than most meats. They have one special benefit: they are free of uric acid. They contain anti-toxic ingredients that help wash the bile while nourishing the gallbladder. Orientals are known for being free of gallbladder difficulties, and their steady diet of soybeans may well be the secret of their health.

SUNFLOWER SEEDS. A good source of polyunsaturated fatty acids, which are needed to liquefy accumulated debris and wash it out of the bile.

Plan to eat a variety of these foods in order to give your gallbladder balanced nutrition and promote healing and revitalization.

SLIM DOWN AND BOOST GALLBLADDER HEALTH

If you are female, overweight, and over 40 years old, you run a greater risk of having gallbladder problems. You may be female and over 40 and still enjoy youthful health . . . if you are *not* fat. Overweight puts a burden on body organs, especially the gallbladder. Overeating forces the gallbladder to strain to produce more and more bile to metabolize excess foods. To help ease the burden of your gallbladder, you should lose excess weight.

How Much Should You Weigh?

The following chart is your guideline. Slimming down is healthful for men and women of any age, so plan to lose weight for the sake of your gallbladder and other organs.

Height (in shoes)	Small Frame		Medium Frame		Large Frame	
	Men	Women	Men	Women	Men	Women
4'10"		95		101		111
5'0"		100		107		117
5'2"	116	106	123	113	133	123
5'4"	122	112	129	119	140	129

Height (in shoes)	Small Frame		Medium Frame		Large Frame	
	Men	Women	Men	Women	Men	Women
5'6"	128	119	136	127	147	137
5'8"	136	127	145	135	156	146
5'10"	145	135	153	143	165	154
6'0"	153	143	162	151	174	163
6'2"	161		171		183	

Tips to Lose Weight and Be Good to Your Gallbladder at the Same Time

As you slim down, you can be good to your gallbladder by following these tips:

1. Eat only very lean meats and limit meat intake to three times a week. Remove all visible fat before cooking and before eating meat.
2. Eat more poultry, except duck and goose.
3. Eat more fish.
4. Prepare foods by baking or broiling. Eliminate fried foods.
5. Use butter and whole dairy products sparingly. Enjoy skim milk, cottage cheese, margarine made from polyunsaturated fats, yogurt, and fermented milk products such as buttermilk.
6. Use liquid oil shortenings or margarine made from polyunsaturated fats for cooking.
7. Cut down on or eliminate bakery products and pastries because they are usually high in saturated fats.
8. Reduce or eliminate refined foods, processed white flour products, and high starch foods.
9. Eat whole grain cereal products and whole grain breads.
10. Eat high fiber fruits and vegetables, raw if possible. Also, drink their juices.

Eliminate "junk" foods, which are low in food value and high in calories. Do not keep prepared foods such as cookies, snacks, and so on in the home. Eat slowly. Reduce the size of your portions. If you get hungry between meals, drink a cup of bouillon or tomato juice or eat low calorie snacks of raw vegetables. If you follow these tips, pounds should start to melt away. At the same time, your gallbladder will be healed and revitalized since it will be relieved of the burden of overweight. Your entire body will respond with rejuvenation and energy. As you slim down, your gallbladder and your other vital organs will improve in health.

HOW CORRECT EATING HABITS HELP HEAL YOUR GALLBLADDER

Because your gallbladder is assigned the task of digesting foods, the way you eat is important for healing and revitalization of this organ. It is as important as what you eat. A healthy gallbladder will empty itself of bile completely about three times during a 24-hour span. To help maintain this pattern, correct and improve your eating methods so that your gallbladder will be able to promote regular rhythmic contractions.

Emotional Health Promotes Gallbladder Health. Eat only when you are emotionally content. Do NOT eat when you are frightened, tired, excited, worried, or nervous. If you do, your gallbladder will contract and *retain* bile fluid instead of transporting it to the duodenum (upper intestine), where it is needed for fat digestion. Do NOT eat when you are emotionally upset. Wait until you feel contented. Your gallbladder will be thankful for your emotional tranquility.

Eat Foods Slowly and Calmly. Chew each mouthful of food leisurely. Swallow only as much as you can comfortably accommodate. Be gentle with your digestive system, and your gallbladder will contract healthfully to send forth fat-digesting bile. Do not gulp down foods. If you are in a hurry, do not eat until you have time to enjoy your food. Do not gulp down beverages, either. Slow, calm eating and drinking will improve the health of your gallbladder.

Foods Should Be at Comfortable Temperatures. Do not shock your gallbladder with an onslaught of foods that are too hot or too cold. Foods and beverages should be at a comfortable temperature to keep your system from being shocked. Your gallbladder will be revitalized through this simple eating tip.

Eat Small Meals Frequently Throughout Day. If you experience gallbladder unrest, soothe this organ by eating smaller meals more often throughout the day. Schedule five smaller meals, two to three hours apart. This matches closely the frequency of emptying rhythms in the gallbladder. Small, frequent meals also guard against over-accumulation of bile.

Protect Yourself from Stress and Tension. Irritability, unrelieved stress, and tension often act upon the gallbladder. They cause unnatural contractions and a backup of bile, which give rise to the "bilious look" or yellowish pallor often noted in nervous people. This is the gallbladder's reaction to prolonged tension. Protect yourself from situations that cause irritating stress and tension. Your gallbladder will be grateful for your emotional tranquility and peacefulness.

Obtain Nightly Rest and Regular Recreation. Be sure to obtain a good night's sleep every night. Refresh yourself with regular recreation and little vacations to ease your emotional and physical stresses. Ordinarily, unrelieved strain brought about by fatigue or sleeplessness "blocks" normal bile flow so that bile backs up into the gallbladder, cholesterol in the bile forms a sediment, and there is the risk of stone accumulation. Protect yourself from this risk with refreshing rest and recreation.

Pamper your gallbladder and improve its health. At the same time, you will be healing and revitalizing all of the related organs. You will then be rewarded with total health and youthful vitality.

IN A NUTSHELL

1. To balance your bile supply and help prevent gallstones, try the doctor's diet for healing and revitalizing the gallbladder.

2. Joan R. corrected painful gallbladder contractions with an everyday food taken before each meal.

3. Andrew MacM. used plant foods and juices to help melt and dissolve gallstones in just three days.

4. Herbal remedies, prepared by a physician, help dissolve gallstones. They are natural prescriptions.

5. Enjoy a variety of everyday foods for healing and revitalization of your gallbladder.

6. Slim down and be good to your gallbladder.

7. Correct your eating methods for improved gallbladder (and body) health.

How to Free Your Stomach
From Ulcer Distress

11

A healthy stomach is the gateway to a revitalized body. When you are able to nourish this digestive organ, your entire body is rewarded with youthful health and vigor. With tasty foods and improved basic body care, you can help protect your stomach from ulcer distress. An ulcer is an open sore. It can interfere with proper digestion and set off a chain reaction whereby the entire body begins to lose health. To guard against this risk and reap the rewards of total revitalization, you need to heal this open sore and improve the health of your stomach.

Ulcer: Causes and Remedies. An ulcer can be caused by body abuse in the form of unrelieved stress and tension, improper foods, emotional and physical irritations such as "knot-like" contractions of the stomach, and faulty eating and living habits.

The most common ulcer is known as the peptic ulcer. There are two types of peptic ulcer: (1) the *duodenal* ulcer is found in the duodenum, that part of the small intestine that lies just outside of the stomach, and (2) the *gastric* ulcer is found in the stomach itself.

More than three million people develop ulcers every year. More than two out of every ten persons will have an ulcer at some time in their lives. Fatalities from ulcers and their complications exceed 12,000 each year.

The basic cause of peptic ulcers can be traced to an excess of gastric juice acting on a damaged mucous membrane of the stomach and actually digesting tissue so as to leave a hole in this membrane and the underlying tissues. An excessive amount of gastric juice (which contains hydrochloric acid) is the underlying cause of ulcer formation.

Stress and tension and unhealthy foods tend to stimulate the vagus nerve, which extends from the brain down the sides of the esophagus to the digestive organs. The vagus nerve then alerts the lower part of the stomach to release gastrin into the bloodstream. Gastrin triggers off the stomach glands to release increased amounts of gastric juice. The stomach cannot cope with this excessive amount of gastric juice and becomes weak and loses resistance. The acid then burns into the tissues of the stomach and a peptic ulcer forms.

Histamine: Substance That Produces Gastric Acid. In particular, histamine (a body substance) powerfully stimulates production of gastric acid. In order to correct and heal ulcer distress, a natural health program is directed toward this basic goal: *block histamine's gastric acid triggering mechanism and "starve" the ulcer so that healing is able to take place.* Or, abolish excess stomach acid and you abolish ulcers!

A physician,[1] Dr. Winea Simpson of the Loma Linda University in California, has prepared a special healing and revitalization program to help heal ulcers. This easy-to-follow program lets you enjoy most of your favorite foods, but it helps control the body mechanism involved in gastric juice production. This program acts as a histamine and gastric juice control to soothe inflammation of the stomach's mucous membranes. It controls the amount of acid that contacts your stomach and helps free your digestive organs from ulcer distress.

STOMACH-REBUILDING, ULCER-HEALING PROGRAM

This program is divided into two parts. The first part involves basic health rules. The second part involves a food program. Follow both of these parts for more effective healing and revitalization of your stomach.

I. Basic Health Rules

Dr. Simpson begins by saying that if you want to help your body build up its own ulcer-healing capability, you must learn to control your emotions. Dr. Simpson offers these basic health rules before presenting the special ulcer-healing diet:

---

[1] "A Diet That Helps Heal Your Ulcer," *Parker Natural Health Bulletin,* West Nyack. New York 10994. February 16, 1976, Vol. 6, No. 4. Available by subscription.

1. Find outlets for supercharged emotions that may set off an ulcer. Emotional upsets may cause damage by increasing stomach acid secretion and by breaking down the resistance of stomach mucous membrane. Weekend diversion, hobbies, and a yearly vacation are important outlets.

2. Learn to live with life and make the most of it. Stop worrying about your work. Get adequate sleep.

3. Eat foods that do not stimulate the secretion of hydrochloric acid and that dilute acid. Vegetable fats such as olive oil, olives, and avocados are especially helpful in controlling acid in the stomach.

4. Olive oil is known to be soothing and protective to the mucous membrane that lines the stomach and intestines. It reduces stomach acid but does not raise blood cholesterol, which makes olive oil preferable to cream as a "coating" for the stomach.

5. Drinking water between meals is important because water dilutes hydrochloric acid. At least six glasses of water a day is a must. The water should not be ice cold, unless it's held in the mouth long enough to warm it.

6. Avoid foods and drugs that stimulate stomach acid, which acts as an irritant to the ulcer. These include sugar-rich foods, coffee, soft drinks, and spicy foods. Also, avoid cigarettes and non-prescription drugs such as aspirin and alkaline powders.

7. Do not take baking soda. It does make the stomach alkaline and does relieve pain, but the aftereffect is irritation of the stomach that causes it to secrete more acid. There is also danger of alkalosis from prolonged use of alkaline powders such as baking soda. Alkaline powders may promote the formation of kidney stones.

8. Establish regular eating habits. Your stomach works rhythmically and needs time to rest. It takes about four hours for a meal to leave the stomach. Eating more often than every four hours doesn't allow time for the stomach to rest.

9. To control both the peak of acidity and deep hunger contractions, eat no more than three moderate meals a day. Eat slowly and chew your food thoroughly. Avoid eating when you are tired, hurried, or emotionally upset.

10. With your doctor's approval, try powdered charcoal (one to two teaspoons) in a glass of water to ease ulcer pain. But this can cause impaction, so use it only with your doctor's guidance.

II. Food Program for Healing of Peptic Ulcer

Dr. Simpson says: "The effect of this food program should be prompt relief of symptoms. Within two to three days, you should be comfortable and free from pain, whether up and about or resting in bed. Failure to gain relief indicates one of three things: incorrect diagnosis, allergy, or complications. If this ulcer program does not bring relief, consult your doctor."

NOTE: Dr. Winea Simpson specifically recommends olive oil at the beginning of each meal to promote healing of the ulcer and to prevent constipation. Three meals a day should be sufficient, but if pain occurs during the night, a glass of skim milk is permissible. Milk mixed with grape juice gives palatable variety.

BREAKFAST

Olive oil, one tablespoon before meal

Milk, one glass, plain or mixed with fruit juice

Cereal, such as rice, Cream of Wheat, and oatmeal

Enriched bread or toast with vegetable oil or margarine

Bland fruit

Raw cashew nuts, two tablespoons, thoroughly chewed or liquified, *or* one egg

LUNCHEON

Olive oil, one tablespoon before meal

Milk, soy milk, or skim milk, one glass

Protein dish such as soy cheese, cottage cheese, Nuteena, and gluten preparation (available at health stores)

Yellow or green vegetable, soft cooked

Starchy food, such a potato, yam, squash, rice, and pureed corn, bake or mash with milk but do not fry

Simple dessert such as cantaloupe

SUPPER

Olive oil, one tablespoon before meal

Cream soup, such as pea, lima bean, rice, and noodle, made with milk or soy milk (available at health store)

Toast or crackers with vegetable margarine

Apricot, prune, or banana whip or stewed bland fruit

Finally, try to maintain a cheerful outlook and concentrate on the pleasant aspects of life. By dwelling on gloomy things rather than happy things, you may produce an ulcer.

THE EVERYDAY VEGETABLE THAT HELPS HEAL STOMACH ULCERS

One everyday vegetable holds the key to solving the problem of stomach ulcers. Cabbage appears to act as a "natural prescription" in healing stomach ulcers. It has been reported[2] by Garnett Cheney, M.D., that *raw cabbage leaves* and *fresh, raw cabbage juice* given to test subjects who had ulcers eliminated the open sores. Dr. Cheney reports that cabbage in the form of raw leaves and juice *protected* against recurrence of the ulcers in test subjects.

Cabbage and Celery Juice Give Freedom from Ulcer Distress. Dr. Cheney treated patients who had ulcers in the duodenum (the eight- to ten-inch length of the alimentary canal that follows the stomach) or had gastric ulcers (in the stomach itself). He prescribed a combination of five ounces of fresh cabbage juice and two ounces of fresh celery juice to be taken five times daily. Juices could be prepared at home with fresh cabbage and celery.

Open Wounds Disappear. Dr. Cheney reported that in 11 out of 13 patients following the cabbage juice and celery juice program, the open wounds disappeared in 6 to 9 days! Dr. Cheney called the mysterious ulcer-healing factor "Vitamin U," the "U" standing for ulcer. Cabbage juice and celery juice form a "natural prescription" that helps heal the stomach and offers freedom from ulcers. These two vegetables, especially in combination, appear to stimulate the body's own defense system to set off an anti-histamine reaction that blocks the acid-triggering mechanism involved in ulcer distress. In-

---

[2] "Healing Ulcers with Cabbages," *California Medicine,* Los Angeles, California, January, 1949, January, 1956.

gredients in both cabbage and celery help shield the stomach and the ulcer from the burning acid and thereby help create healing.

Complete Relief from Ulcer Pain. In another report,[3] a group of 162 ulcer patients was given raw cabbage juice in approximately the same amounts as recommended by Dr. Cheney. As noted by Frederic Damrau, M.D., a medical research consultant who participated: "The results were highly satisfactory. The great majority of patients experienced complete relief from ulcer pain and other subjective complaints after an average of five days on this raw cabbage juice program. Gastric hyperacidity was consistently relieved.

"X-ray examinations showed disappearance of the ulcer niche in 84.6 percent of the patients. After resumption of heavy work for 14 months, relapses occurred in only 12 patients."

How to Use Cabbage Juice as a
Natural Prescription for Ulcer Healing

Effective Cabbages. Dr. Cheney specifies that effective ulcerhealing cabbage juice should be made from cabbage that is fresh, green, and raw. The less time between cabbage picking and consumption, the better. The ulcer-healing ability of the cabbage can be protected through refrigeration of the cabbage until it is ready to be eaten raw or made into juice.

One Quart of Juice Daily. Dr. Cheney's prescription calls for drinking one quart of cabbage juice a day to help heal ulcers already in formation. A smaller amount can protect the stomach from the formation of ulcers.

How to Prepare Juice. Wash some fresh cabbage. Cut it into chunks that can be inserted into opening of your juice maker or grinder. A five pound cabbage will give you one quart of juice, which you can drink throughout the day. (Spring, summer, and late summer cabbages offer more juice. If only winter cabbages are available, you will need twice as many cabbages to produce one quart of juice.) To improve the flavor of the cabbage juice, you may add celery juice (from both the stalks and the greens), citrus juice, pineapple juice, or tomato juice. But you need a minimum of *one quart* of cabbage juice, alone or with other juices. If you have one quart of celery juice, combine it with one quart of cabbage juice and drink the mix-

---

[3] "Ulcer Healing," *Journal of the American Medical Women's Association,* Chicago, Illinois, Vol. 18, No. 6.

ture throughout the day. Other juices may be added according to taste. But you need *one quart of cabbage juice daily.*

To further improve the flavor of the cabbage juice, you may chill it. But do *not* drink it icé cold. It should be comfortably cool for sipping.

Do *not* cook the cabbage juice. Do *not* drink any commercially prepared cabbage juice that has been pasteurized. For the optimum ulcer-healing effect, follow Dr. Cheney's "natural prescription" by squeezing your own cabbage juice and drinking a minimum of one quart each day. This is the natural way to help revitalize your stomach through healing ulcers.

HOW TO "COOL" YOUR "HOT" ULCER IN FIVE MINUTES

The outpouring of gastric acid on the open wound of her ulcer made Lorraine A. feel as if she were "burning up." She wanted to know how to "cool" her "hot," inflamed ulcer in as short a time as possible. She was a dress designer, had to meet many deadlines, and experienced mounting tensions that manifested themselves into an agonizing, scorching pain in her stomach. Lorraine A. had little time or patience for "mind control" class sessions. She wanted to follow some stress-relief program that would offer her fast relief whenever she felt the burning of her hot ulcer. A dress model who attended classroom lessons in biofeedback and mind control told Lorraine A. about a program that included just five steps, one minute for each step. In five minutes, she said, a "hot" ulcer is "cooled." Here is the program that was offered to Lorraine A., who followed it whenever she detected the burning sensation:

1. Make yourself comfortable sitting, standing, or reclining. If possible, be alone or where others cannot distract you.
2. Breathe deeply five times. When you exhale, tell yourself that you are casting out the poisons of stress and tension and "blowing out" toxic and corrosive wastes.
·3. Focus your body weight on the floor beneath you. Visualize all of your weight being lowered and then cast out of your body. Let your physical and mental self "float." Slowly, you will feel your tightness begin to relax and melt away as you feel as light as a fluffy cloud.

4. Let your arms and hands swing idly by your sides. Say to yourself, "I now cast off all negative thoughts, all impure attitudes, all erroneous tensions, and all unhealthy poisons."

5. Shake both hands gently. Visualize all toxic thoughts and physical tensions being washed out of your body through your gently shaking hands onto the ground below.

Each step takes one minute. Together, they take just five minutes. This simple program helped relax the tightness experienced by Lorraine A. It loosened up congestion, transformed negativeness into positiveness, and restored body harmony. Her digestive system was also soothed, and it produced less gastric acid. Her ulcer symptoms slowly subsided. Lorraine A. followed this five-step program several times a day. Within ten days, she was free of the burning sensation. She had revitalized her stomach through simple "thought control" and had eased her ulcer.

HEALING SORE STOMACH WITH PLANTS

Herbs have long been used for healing stomach sores and soothing ulcers. Herbs are available at many health stores and herbal pharmacies. To use them, add 1/4 teaspoon of the powder to a cup of boiled water. You can flavor them with some lemon juice and honey. Drink them as a tea. Several cups taken throughout the day are soothing and beneficial. Folklorists have praised the stomach-healing benefits of these herbs or plants:

ALFALFA. A prime source of digestive enzymes, which break up nutrients and disperse them, thereby guarding against the accumulation of wastes formed by improper metabolism. This process helps cleanse the stomach tract, soothe open sores, and promote better healing.

COMFREY. When comfrey is brewed as a tea, the boiled liquid releases *allantoin,* a nitrogenous crystalline substance that acts as a cell proliferant. That is, the allantoin boosts the healing of the cells and tissues that have become raw and inflamed due to an ulcer. Allantoin in the comfrey plant acts as a healer that binds the cells together to free the stomach of ulcer problems.

LICORICE. Use the natural herb instead of the synthetic candy. When it is boiled and used as a tea, it releases an estrogenic material that acts as a demulcent and emollient for the digestive tract. That is, the estrogenic material is somewhat oily and coats the abraded mucous membrane to protect it against irritation. It also softens and smooths the surface so that there is less abrasion and irritation. Drink licorice tea regularly for this stomach revitalizing benefit.

SLIPPERY ELM. When it is brewed as a tea, the inner bark of slippery elm releases an emollient that soothes inflamed ulcers, helping to cool them and provide needed relief from the burning sensation. Make the tea as thick as possible for better coating action upon the open sore to promote swifter healing.

To help heal and revitalize the stomach, use these herb teas regularly whenever you need a beverage.

THE GRAIN FOOD THAT CONTROLS STOMACH ACID AND HEALS ULCERS

An everyday grain food that costs just pennies per average serving can help control stomach acid. This simple grain food, available just about everywhere, acts as a natural barrier to excess acid. It *shields* and *insulates* the stomach against the onrush of burning acid that can scorch the mucous membrane and pave the way for agonizing ulcer distress. This everyday grain food is *fiber.*

What Is It? Fiber, also known as bran and roughage, is the outer coating of whole grains, such as wheat germ, corn, whole grain cereals, and rye, fibrous vegetables, such as carrots, celery, parsnips, and squash, and fruits, such as apricots, apples, blackberries, dates, and raspberries. For the most part, however, fiber is found in *unrefined grain foods.*

How Fiber Blocks Excess Acid Flow. Stress or no stress, an internal "conflict" rages between the natural secretions of the stomach. First, the stomach releases hydrochloric acid and pepsin, which are used to digest food. Then, the stomach releases mucin as a coating to protect itself from being digested. A problem exists if the amount of hydrochloric acid and pepsin increases and disturbs the acid-pepsin/mucin balance. The stomach becomes open to attack from its own secretions. This predisposes the stomach to ulcer formation. This problem can be averted with sufficient fiber in the daily diet.

Fiber acts as a *natural buffering agent* to protect the stomach from an excess of hydrochloric acid and pepsin in the system. *Fiber contains protein, which neutralizes hydrochloric acid and pepsin so that the mucin coating can resist burning.*

To ease ulcer pain and block excess acid flow, eat high-protein fiber foods daily.

Ends Stomach Burning and Eliminates Ulcer Trouble. Walter T. C. blamed his "acid stomach" and burning ulcer on his stressful job as a construction supervisor. Yet when he was transferred to a comparatively tension-free desk job, Walter T. C. still felt the agonizing churning and the burning sensation that reached right up into his throat. So he realized that stress and tension are not always the cause of stomach burning and ulcer pain. He discussed his problem with a nutrition scientist, who told him that he needed to boost his protein-containing fiber intake as a way of building resistance to acid attack on his stomach. Here is the program outlined for Walter T. C.:

Basic Program: Every day, plan to take eight tablespoons of pure, unprocessed bran. This grain is available in all health stores and many food markets.

1. *Breakfast.* Take two tablespoons of bran mixed with scrambled eggs, with any whole grain cereal and fruit and milk, or with waffles, pancakes, or French toast.

2. *Noon.* Add two tablespoons of bran to any clear soup, sprinkle it over a raw fruit or vegetable salad as part of the dressing, mix it with any baked dish, or dissolve it in several cups of herb tea or fruit or vegetable juice.

3. *Evening.* Add two tablespoons of bran to any baked meat loaf, casserole, chowder, or main dish. Sprinkle it over a raw fruit or vegetable salad.

4. *Snack.* Add two tablespoons of bran to a cup of plain or fruit-flavored yogurt, or add them to a cup of cottage cheese. Stir bran into any sugar-free custard or fruit cocktail.

Benefits of Bran Program. The eight tablespoons of pure, unprocessed bran boostered Walter T. C.'s protein intake. The protein offered a natural buffering action by neutralizing the hydrochloric acid and pepsin. The protein-rich bran helped keep the acid/pepsin-mucin ratio at a non-ulcerous level. Walter T. C. found relief from his constant stomach burning. The ulcer pain ended. Soon, he found freedom from the threat of ulcer flare-up and could return to his stressful job as a construction supervisor with a happy stomach, happy body and, happy mind.

ELIMINATE REFINED FOODS FOR REVITALIZED STOMACH HEALTH

To control acid flow, eliminate refined foods from your diet. These bleached and "stripped" foods have had their valuable protein partially or completely removed. With little or no protein, refined foods cannot neutralize hydrochloric acid and pepsin. When refined foods enter the digestive tract, the lining of the stomach is exposed to acid because of the lack of sufficient protein. Repeated intake of refined foods may pave the way for recurring ulcer problems.

Note: "Enrichment" puts back some of the vitamins and minerals but not fiber. Avoid enriched foods, except where absolutely necessary or in the absence of wholesome foods. To compensate for the loss of important protein-containing fiber, plan to eat at least eight tablespoons of pure bran daily, throughout the day, with cooked foods and beverages. It is the "natural" ulcer healer!

Eliminate These Stomach Offenders: Eliminate *coffee and soft drinks* because these contain caffeine, which acts as an acid-stimulating agent and causes an outpouring of this burning fluid onto the stomach. Eliminate *tobacco* because smoking constricts blood vessels to hinder the free flow of needed mucin for coating the stomach and thereby renders the stomach vulnerable to acid burning. Eliminate *alcoholic beverages* because they cause sporadic opening and closing of the blood vessels, and the resulting erratic spurts of acid and mucin cause internal upset and stomach distress. By eliminating these stomach offenders, you will help heal and revitalize your vital digestive organs and offer natural protection from ulcer problems.

IN REVIEW

1. To help control and buffer the hydrochloric acid that causes stomach problems, follow the doctor-created Stomach-Rebuilding, Ulcer-Healing Program.

2. Use one tablespoon of olive oil before each meal to coat the stomach and help protect it against the burning of stomach acid.

3. An everyday vegetable and its raw juice helped heal ulcers in a doctor-supervised program that can be followed at home.

4. Lorraine A. learned to "cool" her "hot" ulcer in five minutes with an easy relaxation program.

5. Heal a sore stomach with a variety of herbs prepared as delicious teas.

6. An everyday grain food is a prime source of protein, which can help control stomach acid and heal ulcers.

7. Walter T. C. ended stomach burning and ulcer trouble by taking eight tablespoons of pure bran throughout the day.

8. Eliminate refined foods and the stomach offenders listed in this chapter for greater digestive health and freedom from ulcer problems.

Rebuilding Your Respiratory Organs
For Refreshing Rejuvenation

12

You can live for weeks without food and for days without water, but you can survive for only a few moments without air. Oxygen is needed for metabolizing nutrients that are transported via your bloodstream to all parts of your body. While food and water can be stored in your body, oxygen cannot. That is why you must breathe constantly. You must oxygenate your body through "total breathing" so that your billions of cells and tissues become adequately nourished. With an abundance of nutrients, your vital organs can be rebuilt to help provide your entire body with a feeling of refreshing rejuvenation.

HOW TO HEAL BRONCHIAL DISORDERS BY "PAYING OFF" YOUR "OXYGEN DEBT"

Nancy H. developed breathing difficulties in her middle years. She would awaken in the middle of the night with coughing spasms. At times, she had such tight chest constrictions that she would wheeze, sputter, and turn pale as she staggered to an open window to try to take in some precious air. She blamed it on her "age" even though she was hardly into her 60's. Nancy H. also started to look pale and developed crow's feet around her eyes. She often walked with a stooped gait. She resigned herself to worsening bronchial trouble. Medications made her nauseous. Patent remedies also gave her an upset stomach, and they did little to relieve her condition. She felt miserable.

153

Simple "No Work" Exercise Rejuvenates Respiratory Organs.
Nancy H. might have suffered in choked silence had not a neighboring physiotherapist come to her rescue. He said that she needed to
correct the *cause* of her respiratory organ breakdown. The *cause* was
an "oxygen debt." Years of sedentary living had caused a gradual
decrease in the levels of oxygen in her respiratory organs. Choked for
air and starved for nutrients, which are transported by the oxygen-
nourished bloodstream, her organs were weakening, "aging," and
reacting through bronchial problems. She needed to "pay off" her
oxygen debt through a simple "no work" exercise program. The
physiotherapist told Nancy H. that an effortless exercise would increase her respiratory activity and provide pulmonary ventilation
that would saturate her organs with nourishing oxygen. She could
thereby settle her oxygen debt and refresh and rejuvenate her respiratory system.

Program: The physiotherapist told Nancy H. to walk up a hill or
a flight of stairs *leisurely* and *slowly*, without any strain. He told her
to do this for ten minutes in the morning and ten minutes in the
evening. Every day for seven days, Nancy H. had to increase her
walking time by about five minutes each walk. She was told that by
the end of seven days she should be able to do this easy exercise for
about 40 minutes each session. Nancy H. followed the program for
seven days. Slowly, her breathing improved. By the end of the seven
days, she was breathing as she did when she was a child. Gone were
the nightly coughing spells. She felt no tightness in her chest. Her
face regained its color. Her posture was youthfully erect. Her bronchial disorders were a thing of the past.

To help keep her respiratory organs in their new youthful condition, Nancy H. continued to walk uphill or upstairs as often as was
comfortably possible throughout the week. This program is the "no
cost" and "no effort" way to rebuild respiratory organs.

Benefits of Repaying an Oxygen Debt. The respiratory organs
require exercise like other organs. If they are allowed to become
lazy, they lose their capacity to transport sufficient oxygen, and not
only the bronchial system but all other body organs start to falter.
The respiratory organs, choked for air, build up the "oxygen debt,"
and the health of the whole body suffers.

Walking uphill or upstairs helps exercise the respiratory organs.
This easy motion sends a stream of valuable oxygen through the
respiratory organs to the other body organs for overall nourishment.
The benefits include:

1. There is an increase in size of the respiratory organs, which improves breathing and protects them from bronchial wheezing.

2. Lung capillaries increase in size and number during uphill walking. This enables more oxygen to be absorbed by the respiratory and other body organs.

3. Lung capacity is increased and more oxygen can be inhaled so that the oxygen debt is speedily repaid.

4. The alveoli (air sacs) become more functional so that there is a greater transfer of oxygen and carbon dioxide. This permits better body ventilation.

5. The rate of breathing improves and *deeper* respiration occurs so that oxygen can be sent to the most distant portions of the respiratory organs.

Oxygen-washed respiratory organs can function more vigorously and send nutrients to other organs to help keep them refreshingly rejuvenated.

All you have to do is walk *uphill* or *upstairs* whenever possible as an easy way to exercise your respiratory organs and boost basic body health. That way, you'll repay your oxygen debt and bank on youthful vitality.

HOW "BABY BREATHING" CAN HELP KEEP YOU YOUNG

Gloria D. had to gasp for air upon the slightest exertion. She had a nervous twitch. At times, her hands and head shook like those of a person with a muscular-nervous ailment. She complained that her lungs were so "choked" that she could hardly say more than a few words at a time without having to stop for breath. When she slept, her breathing was a wheeze like that of an elderly person. Gloria D. coughed frequently. She had an ashen skin that developed premature wrinkles. She tried various patent remedies, but they made her groggy and dizzy and distorted her vision. So she eagerly listened as a local lecturer told how "baby breathing" could promote total body rejuvenation.

Basic Benefit: Baby breathing is abdominal or "belly breathing." Note how a baby breathes this way. Perhaps it is nature's suggestion that this type of breathing offers hope for respiratory and total body rejuvenation. Baby breathing uses the belly and diaphragm. It is more refreshing than regular breathing because it fills the lungs completely with each inhalation and empties the lungs with each exhalation. *Retaining the inhaled breath allows incoming air to purify the bloodstream, which is not possible with shallow or ordinary breathing.*

"Belly Breathing" Is More Rejuvenating Than "Thorax Breathing." "Belly breathing" sends bloodstream-washing air throughout the respiratory organs to cleanse them and free them of toxic wastes. Ordinary "thorax breathing" (the thorax is the region from the neck to the abdomen in the chest) consists of short, *shallow* breaths. It retains stale air in the lungs. The lungs become oxygen-starved and begin to falter in function. When you follow a "belly breathing" technique, which is similar to that of "baby breathing," you send rejuvenating oxygen throughout your organs and are rewarded with youthful health.

Technique: Lie down on the floor (use a large towel or blanket as a mat). Put your hands gently on your abdomen, just below your navel, or belly button. Let your fingertips touch. Now follow these steps:

1. Inhale through your nose and simultaneously let your belly swell out like a "pot belly." Let your fingertips part as your belly swells out. Inhale very deeply.

2. Exhale through your nose and simultaneously pull in your stomach so that your fingertips touch again. Suck in your stomach as you exhale.

Do these easy "belly breathing" techniques up to ten times daily.

Refreshes and Rejuvenates Respiratory Organs. This simple program is able to refresh and rejuvenate more than just the respiratory organs; it refreshes the entire body. It improves blood pressure, opens the blood vessels leading to the heart, and nourishes and tones up the entire neurological system. It fills the torso with oxygen. It washes out the system and cleans it of accumulated wastes that can cause premature aging.

Feels "Forever Young" with "Belly Breathing" Technique. Gloria D. followed this simple technique every morning and every night for two weeks. She felt her lungs improving. She no longer gasped for breath. Her skin became pink and healthy. She became so active that she wanted a part-time job in addition to her regular family housekeeping duties. She continues doing the "belly breathing" technique at least once a day, and thanks to her rejuvenated respiratory organs she feels young again.

HOW "STRETCH HEALING" REVITALIZES RESPIRATORY ORGANS

Improve your thinking capacities and tap the hidden reserves of youthful alertness through "stretch healing." When you follow this simple program, you send a flood of oxygen through your respiratory organs and to your brain. Your billions of brain cells receive important oxygen. When the respiratory center of your brain receives stimuli informing it of a need for oxygen, it sends nerve impulses to your chest muscles, which cause alternate inhalation and exhalation. This causes a gaseous exchange between the alveoli (air sacs) and your bloodstream. Your brain benefits from this exchange and reacts with more youthful alertness and vigor.

"Stretch healing" helps loosen congestion in your body to permit free exchange of oxygen between the respiratory organs and the brain.

Three Steps to Simple "Stretch Healing"

1. In a quiet environment, sit down in a chair. Close your eyes. Visualize tension spots in various parts of your body: face muscles, shoulders, chest, stomach, and so on. Then visualize yourself relaxing these muscles since they are channels through which your respiratory organs will transport needed oxygen.

2. With your eyes still closed, stand up. Now, very slowly and deliberately, stretch. Visualize a cat streching. Do it luxuriously, enjoyably. Reach for the ceiling with both hands. Just stretch and stretch and stretch. Do NOT strain. Visualize a cat that *never* strains when stretching but just immerses itself in the sheer joy of indulgent stretching. Do the same. As you stretch and reach upward, breathe in and out very deeply. You should feel tension being washed out with each exhalation.

3. Now sigh. Exhale. Sit down. Feel yourself relax. Open your eyes after several minutes.

Benefits: This "stretch healing" relaxes knots, permits a freer exchange of oxygen and carbon dioxide, and sends a stream of oxygen to the brain so that there is improved mental power. If you are occupied with a task in which you must hold your head over a table or desk, looking at papers or other items for long periods of time, you are placing severe tension on the muscles of your neck and shoulders. Congestion will deprive your brain of needed oxygen. Enjoy "stretch healing" as a break during any prolonged mental work, and you will feel your brain becoming refreshed. You will then be able to return to your work with greater mental and physical vigor.

HOW TO "PULSE BREATHE" YOUR WAY TO YOUTHFUL HEALTH

Theodore J. erupted in an asthmatic choking spasm whenever he became nervous. He would often find himself sputtering and gasping when he tried to doze off or take a nap. He had tried chemicalized vaporizers, but they only offered momentary relief and did not end his problem of "aged" lungs. He maintained that he was getting old before his time because of this sputtering and choking and was resigned to this fate.

One day he happened to attend a local yoga demonstration with his wife, and that was when he discovered that a "pulse breathing" program would restore his lungs to youthful health. Theodore J. followed this program, three times a day for two weeks. Slowly, his asthmatic attacks subsided and his breathing improved. He felt youthfully alert and vigorous.

Basic "Pulse Breathing" Technique: Maintain a comfortable sitting position. If possible, sit cross-legged on the floor. Press the thumb of one hand on the inside of the opposite wrist, keeping the fingers on the outside of that wrist just as a doctor does when he takes your pulse.

When you can feel your pulse, inhale for a count of ten pulse beats. Then hold your breath for the count of two pulse beats. Then exhale for the count of ten pulse beats.

Tip: As you follow this easy "pulse breathing" technique, close your eyes and visualize a fresh air country scene. This will help soothe your tension spots and open channels through which more nourishing oxygen may travel to all parts of your body.

"Pulse breathing" does more than strengthen the respiratory organs. It perks up all of the organs and systems in your body and promotes a feeling of total rejuvenation. In just five minutes, you can supercharge your body with this easy, enjoyable, and effortless technique. If offers a life of healthy revitalization!

HOME REMEDIES FOR RESPIRATORY ORGAN DISORDERS

Follow these home remedies to boost the health of your respiratory organs so that you can overcome respiratory disorders.

COLDS. Strengthen the cold-fighting powers of the mucous membranes of your nostrils by drinking lots of citrus juices for Vitamin C. This vitamin builds up the membrane integrity so that germs cannot invade the body so easily. *Always* breathe through your nose when you are out in chilly weather to filter out harmful organisms. If the air is unusually cold, hold a clean handkerchief to your nose and warm the air before you inhale it.

SINUS DISTRESS. Eliminate table salt from your diet. Table salt tends to constrict nasal tissues and appears to predispose you to suffering a sinus attack. Eliminate all refined starches and sugars since they use up the body's supply of vitamins to make you more susceptible to sinus, nasal passage, and chest congestions. Follow the inhalation therapies in this chapter to help cleanse your bloodstream of toxic wastes that could trigger off sinus attacks.

BRONCHITIS. Keep your entire body warm. Go on a special liquid food fast in which solids are avoided and fresh liquids are taken throughout the day. A liquid food fast helps wash out accumulated toxic wastes from your system and ease congestion in the nose, throat, and chest areas. Inhale warm air only. Avoid temperature extremes in air that you breathe and in food that you eat.

COUGHS. A folklore healer calls for boiling whole grain oats in as little water as possible to make a mash. Flavor the mash with a bit of honey and eat it with a spoon. Ingredients in the oats such as polyunsaturated fatty acids appear to soothe inflammation of the bronchial region and respiratory organs to offer relief from coughing spasms. Take this *oat mash* throughout the day. It should always be comfortably warm. Folklorists prescribe one cup at a time.

CHEST PAINS. Ease chest congestion with a simple hot water pack. Soak a flannel cloth in hot water. Take care not to burn your hands. When the cloth is comfortable to the touch, fold it to a comfortable thickness and place it against your chest between the nipples. Leave it on until it is cool. Repeat this procedure several times. The warmth of the cloth seeps through the pores of your skin and soothes spasms to give relief from chest pains.

SHORT BREATH. Shortness of breath is often accompanied by digestive aches, which indicate that the body organs are closely related to one another so that if one is malfunctioning the others feel the effect. To correct shortness of breath, follow this simple breathing exercise: Sit comfortably. Push out your stomach when you inhale. Suck in your stomach when you exhale. Inhale and exhale like this ten times. This helps nourish your parched lungs. At the same time, the rhythmic motion helps loosen accumulated wastes and cleanse your digestive system so that you can breathe healthfully and your stomach is free from pains.

MORNING CONGESTION. Many people awaken in the morning after a good night's sleep and experience chest tightness and sniffles. These problems may be traced to breathing cold night air. To protect yourself against these problems, tie a clean handkerchief loosely around your nose before you retire for the night. Make sure that it does not restrict normal night movements. The handkerchief will *warm* air as it is inhaled so that respiratory organs are not chilled in the night. You will awaken feeling comfortable and without the irritating chest congestion caused by hours of cold air inhalation during sleep.

Breath is life! Revitalize your respiratory organs with easy breathing techniques. Whenever possible, get out into the fresh and pollution-free countryside. Fresh air warms quicker than air that has been diluted or comes from an artificial source such as an air conditioner. Indoor air is stale air. It lacks the important elements found in fresh and pollution-free air. Schedule countryside or oceanside trips regularly and drink deeply of nature's respiratory organ tonic—fresh air, the elixir of youthful health.

HIGHLIGHTS

1. Nancy H. healed bronchial disorders by paying off her oxygen debt with an easy "no work" exercise.
2. Gloria D. felt young again through simple "baby breathing" techniques.

3. "Stretch healing" helps revitalize the respiratory organs and all other organs.

4. Theodore J. "pulse breathed" his way to youthful health in a few minutes and corrected his asthmatic disorders.

5. Ease and eliminate respiratory organ disorders with a variety of easy-to-follow home remedies.

How to Activate, Alert, and Amplify Your Pancreas for Improved Metabolism

13

Enjoy more vim and vigor, feel more energetic throughout the day, and radiate the joy of living through an alert *pancreas*. The pancreas is a little-known but highly important organ that sends hormone messengers throughout your body, influences food metabolism, and has the power to make you feel youthful, alert, and emotionally happy. A healthy pancreas creates a happy body!

Location of Pancreas. The pancreas is situated behind the lower part of the stomach. It is a large gland. It is broadest on the right, where it nestles in the curve of the duodenum (first part of the stomach), wrapped around the portal vein and closely applied to the arteries of the liver and the bile duct. At this point, it tapers away, upward and to the left, between the stomach and the left kidney to reach the spleen. The pancreas is part of this network of organs. It must be properly nourished and cared for in order to provide your body with important metabolic hormones and digestive juices.

Function of Pancreas. As part of the digestive system, the pancreas releases a pancreatic juice into the intestines to work with other digestive juices in breaking down food into nutrients that can be used to heal, rebuild, and revitalize your entire body.

Pancreas Regulates Blood Sugar. One important function of the pancreas is to regulate the levels of sugar in the blood. A *balanced blood sugar* can give you youthful vitality, emotional alertness, healthy vigor, and a feeling of limitless energy. The pancreas is in charge of balancing your blood sugar level to give you this feeling of mind and body vitality. One small section of the pancreas, called the islets of Langerhans, is in charge of this energy-boosting job. A healthy pancreas can boost your feelings of vitality through a balanced blood sugar level.

Pancreas Protects You from Diabetes. The pancreas produces a hormone called *insulin.* (A hormone is a substance released by a gland that influences the activity of other glands and organs.) Insulin is the spark that ignites the fire for the burning of sugars and starches to transform them into youthful energy and body warmth. The result of a poorly functioning pancreas is insufficient burning of sugar. The excess sugar flows into the urine after the blood has become saturated with it. This condition is known as diabetes. In diabetes the pancreas fails to create sufficient amounts of insulin for sugar and starch burning. A healthy pancreas producing a healthy supply of insulin is the best protection against diabetes.

HOW REFINED SUGAR CAN WEAKEN THE PANCREAS

To improve and strengthen the health of your pancreas, you should eliminate refined sugar in all of its forms from your diet. When your body takes in refined sugar, the islets of Langerhans must work harder to handle the overload. These pancreatic cells work furiously to release insulin to metabolize the refined sugar. An overload of refined sugar can cause such an overworking of the islets of Langerhans that the entire pancreas will become exhausted. When this organ is weak, it falters in its release of sugar-metabolizing insulin, leading to the double threat of low blood sugar (hypoglycemia) and diabetes. Refined sugar abuses the pancreas, and it should be eliminated from your diet

ELIMINATE REFINED SUGAR FROM KITCHEN

To heal and revitalize your pancreas and protect yourself from erratic blood sugar levels and diabetes, eliminate refined sugar from your kitchen. Do not use it to sweeten any food or beverage, fresh or cooked. Do not keep any refined sugar in your house. Replace it with honey, blackstrap molasses, pure maple syrup, and date powder. These are available in many supermarkets and health food stores. Use them moderately since they are high in calories. You should avoid using these natural sugars in any excessive amount. They also need to be metabolized by the pancreas, and you should not overburden this organ with an excessive amount of sugar in your system.

You should restrict or eliminate any packaged foods containing refined sugar. The following chart will show you how much refined sugar is found in many everyday foods.

So you think you don't eat much sugar?

Here are the approximate amounts of refined sugar
(added sugar, in addition to the sugar naturally present)
hidden in popular foods.

Food item	Size Portion	Approximate Sugar Content in Teaspoonful of Granulated Sugar
Beverages		
cola drinks	1 (6 oz bottle or glass)	3 1/2
cordials	1 (3/4 oz glass)	1 1/2
ginger ale	6 oz	5
highball	1 (6 oz glass)	2 1/2
orangeade	1 (8 oz glass)	5
root beer	1 (10 oz bottle)	4 1/2
Seven-Up®	1 (6 oz bottle or glass)	3 3/4
soda pop	1 (8 oz bottle)	5
sweet cider	1 cup	6
whiskey sour	1 (3 oz glass)	1 1/2
Cakes and Cookies		
angel food	1 (4 oz piece)	7
apple sauce cake	1 (4 oz piece)	5 1/2
banana cake	1 (2 oz piece)	2
cheese cake	1 (4 oz piece)	2
chocolate cake (plain)	1 (4 oz piece)	6
chocolate cake (iced)	1 (4 oz piece)	10
coffee cake	1 (4 oz piece)	4 1/2
cup cake (iced)	1	6
fruit cake	1 (4 oz piece)	5
jelly roll	1 (2 oz piece)	2 1/2
orange cake	1 (4 oz piece)	4
pound cake	1 (4 oz piece)	5
sponge cake	1 (1 oz piece)	2
brownies (unfrosted)	1 (3/4 oz)	3
chocolate cookies	1	1 1/2
Fig Newtons®	1	5
gingersnaps	1	3
macaroons	1	6
nut cookies	1	1 1/2

Food item	Size Portion	Approximate Sugar Content in Teaspoonful of Granulated Sugar
oatmeal cookies	1	2
sugar cookies	1	1 1/2
chocolate eclair	1	7
cream puff	1	2
donut (plain)	1	3
donut (glazed)	1	6
Candies		
average chocolate milk bar	1 (1 1/2 oz)	2 1/2
chewing gum	1 stick	1/2
chocolate cream	1 piece	2
butterscotch chew	1 piece	1
chocolate mints	1 piece	2
fudge	1 oz square	4 1/2
gumdrop	1	2
hard candy	4 oz	20
Lifesavers®	1	1/3
peanut brittle	1 oz	3 1/2
Canned Fruits and Juices		
canned apricots	4 halves and 1 T syrup	3 1/2
canned fruit juices (sweet)	1/2 cup	2
canned peaches	2 halves and 1 T syrup	3 1/2
fruit salad	1/2 cup	3 1/2
fruit syrup	2 T	2 1/2
stewed fruits	1/2 cup	2
Dairy Products		
ice cream	1/3 pt (3 1/2 oz)	3 1/2
ice cream cone	1	3 1/2
ice cream soda	1	5
ice cream sundae	1	7
malted milk shake	1 (10 oz glass)	5
Jams and Jellies		
apple butter	1 T	1
jelly	1 T	4–6
orange marmalade	1 T	4–6
peach butter	1 T	1
strawberry jam	1 T	4
Desserts, Miscellaneous		
apple cobbler	1/2 cup	3
blueberry cobbler	1/2 cup	3
custard	1/2 cup	2
french pastry	1 (4 oz piece)	5
fruit gelatin	1/2 cup	4 1/2
apple pie	1 slice (average)	7
apricot pie	1 slice	7
berry pie	1 slice	10
butterscotch pie	1 slice	4

Food Item	Size Portion	Approximate Sugar Content in Teaspoonful of Granulated Sugar
cherry pie	1 slice	10
cream pie	1 slice	4
lemon pie	1 slice	7
mince meat pie	1 slice	4
peach pie	1 slice	7
prune pie	1 slice	6
pumpkin pie	1 slice	5
rhubarb pie	1 slice	4
banana pudding	1/2 cup	2
bread pudding	1/2 cup	1 1/2
chocolate pudding	1/2 cup	4
cornstarch pudding	1/2 cup	2 1/2
date pudding	1/2 cup	7
fig pudding	1/2 cup	7
Grapenut® pudding	1/2 cup	2
plum pudding	1/2 cup	4
rice pudding	1/2 cup	5
tapioca pudding	1/2 cup	3
berry tart	1 cup	10
blancmange	1/2 cup	5
brown Betty	1/2 cup	3
plain pastry	1 (4 oz piece)	3
sherbet	1/2 cup	9
Syrups, Sugars, and Icings		
brown sugar	1 T	*3
chocolate icing	1 oz	5
chocolate sauce	1 T	3 1/2
corn syrup	1 T	*3
granulated sugar	1 T	*3
honey	1 T	*3
Karo® syrup	1 T	*3
maple syrup	1 T	*5
molasses	1 T	*3 1/2
white icing	1 oz	*5

*actual sugar content

A PANCREAS-HEALING FOOD PROGRAM
FOR TOTAL REJUVENATION

Arlene Q. was a "sugar-holic." She not only liked to snack on candies and cookies, but she also used several heaping tablespoons of refined sugar in a cup of coffee or tea. This excess sugar overburdened her pancreas, which had to work doubly hard to accommodate the onrush of refined sugar. Consequently, Arlene Q. began to experience symptoms of hypoglycemia. Her hands trembled. She was energetic for a few moments and then suddenly felt exhausted. She stumbled over words. Her memory was fuzzy. She seemed confused. Tests showed that she had too much sugar in her urine. This was a clue that her overburdened pancreas could not release enough sugar-metabolizing insulin. Arlene Q. was told by a nutrition specialist that she would have to "kick" the sugar habit and follow a food program that would heal and revitalize her pancreas in order to find relief from her health problems. Here is the tasty program she followed:

Trim Overweight. Excess pounds overwork most body organs, especially the pancreas, which is involved in metabolizing calorie-filled sugars and starches. To rebuild the pancreas, trim unwanted and unnecessary pounds.

Avoid All Refined Carbohydrates. Eliminate foods listed on the sugar chart. These are refined foods, which have been stripped of vitamins, minerals, and proteins needed to nourish the pancreas. Switch to whole grain cereals, fresh fruits, and fresh vegetables, raw or cooked but without refined sugar.

Enjoy Sweetbread. Sweetbread is an animal's pancreas. Enjoy it baked or broiled in a bit of vegetable oil. It is a good supply of the mineral zinc, which is found in high concentrations in the hormone insulin. By nourishing your pancreas with zinc from sweetbreads, you help give it strength and power. You promote its insulin-making power through zinc nourishment. Sweetbreads, available at your local butcher, are a healthy and tasty pancreas-rebuilding food.

Vitamins from Whole Grain Foods Help Lower Sugar Levels. The B-complex vitamins (niacin, riboflavin, pantothenic acid, and pyridoxine) are especially powerful in helping to "dissolve" excess sugar in the bloodstream. They are plentiful in whole grain breads, cereals, wheat germ, bran, brewer's yeast, broiled and baked liver, and desiccated liver. These products are available in most supermarkets and health stores. Eat them regularly.

The Healthy Sweet for Your Pancreas (and Sweet Tooth). Your pancreas will benefit from a healthy sweet found in fresh fruits. Your "sweet tooth" will find satisfaction in the *natural* and *unrefined* sweetness of most fresh fruits. Select *tart* fruits, such as cranberries and cranberry juice, grapefruit, various berries, and most other fruits. *Benefit:* Much of the fruit's sugar (especially in tart fruits) is in the form of fructose, which requires almost no insulin for its metabolism in the body's cells. (Some fructose is transformed into glucose for storage before it leaves the digestive system, so do not eat it in a concentrated form.) Tart fruits nourish your pancreatic cells without any burdensome metabolic requirements. Eat fresh fruit regularly for rebuilding your pancreas and satisfaction of your sweet tooth.

Cold-Pressed Oils for Better Sugar Metabolism. Cold-pressed oils are available at most supermarkets and health stores. Cold-pressed oils are naturally pressed seed and vegetable oils. No heat is used in processing, which helps preserve the perishable vitamins and essential fatty acids. In particular, cold-pressed oils (soy, sesame, safflower, wheat germ, corn, and others) contain Vitamin E, which promotes sugar metabolism and storage in the muscles. This improves basic blood circulation, an essential benefit for people with weak pancreases who fear the development of diabetes. Use cold-pressed oils with a bit of lemon juice or apple cider vinegar on raw vegetable salads.

Fish Liver Oils for More Vitamins. Use cod liver oil, shark liver oil, and other oils from fish livers to help nourish your pancreas with Vitamin A. While vegetables contain a precursor (a substance that is transformed into Vitamin A by your system) of Vitamin A, if your pancreas is weak it cannot convert the precursor, or "carotene," into Vitamin A. Boost pancreatic health with fish liver oils (take up to six tablespoons daily, mixed with a fruit juice if you like). Continue eating raw vegetables for other nutrients.

Boost Potassium Intake for Pancreas Power. A weak pancreas may lead to diabetes and potassium loss. Potassium is needed to nourish and invigorate the pancreas. Boost your potassium intake through daily intake of bananas, oranges, pineapples, pecans, buckwheat, and navy beans. Eat these foods regularly to supply potassium to your pancreas.

Balances Blood Sugar and Erases Threat of Diabetes. Arlene Q. followed this tasty program for no more than three weeks. Almost from the start, she felt an improvement. Her once-trembling hands were now as steady as those of a youngster. She felt youthful energy from morning until late in the evening. Her speech and memory became sharp and alert. She no longer seemed confused and "lost." The Pancreas-Healing Food Program strengthened her important body organ. Her blood sugar was balanced. Her doctor told her the threat of diabetes was erased. Life became cheerful and beautiful for Arlene Q.

THE SWEET FOOD THAT DISSOLVES EXCESS SUGAR IN THE BLOODSTREAM

Laurence O' D. was examined by his company doctor and was told that he showed symptoms of too much sugar in his bloodstream. He was nervous about developing diabetes since his family had a history of this ailment. Laurence O' D. did not like drugs because they made him dizzy. Sometimes he felt as if he were going to faint. So he wanted a natural way to help dissolve the excess sugar in his bloodstream. He asked the doctor about natural remedies and was told to try the following easy program, which involved a sweet food. He could have this sweet and enjoy it while it dissolved the excess sugar in his bloodstream.

Blueberries and Their Leaves: Every day, Laurence O' D. ate a pint or more of fresh blueberries. He was allowed to flavor them with a bit of honey. If fresh blueberries were unavailable, he was allowed to eat frozen blueberries provided the package label said that there was no sugar added. Laurence O' D. also used blueberry leaves (available at herbal pharmacies and many health stores) to make a tea. He let one or two leaves brew in a cup or more of boiling water. He added a slice of lemon and a bit of honey for flavor.

Benefits: Blueberries and blueberry leaves contain a natural substance known as *myrtillin.* This is a "plant hormone" that acts to help dissolve sugar in the bloodstream. *Myrtillin* is considered a "natural insulin" because of its sugar-dissolving abilities. It also helps stablize blood sugar. American Indians, who ate blueberries and brewed the blueberry leaves to make a tea, were generally free of diabetes. They may have protected themselves against diabetes through the *myrtillin* they ingested.

Recovers from Sugar Problem. Laurence O' D. followed this simple and sweet program. He also eliminated refined sugar from his diet. After three weeks, his company doctor tested him and reported that he no longer had any sugar overload. Laurence O' D., who had a family history of diabetes, had revitalized his pancreas with the blueberry program. It was as sweet as it was healthful!

REBUILDING THE PANCREAS ON A TWO-DAY HIGH-MINERAL FAST

To heal and revitalize the health of your pancreas, go on a two-day high-mineral fast. When your body is overburdened with acid because of over-indulgence in refined sugars and starches, your pancreas reacts by pouring out more insulin. Your pancreas is overworked, and as it weakens it releases less insulin. This leads to an over-accumulation of sugar. To help rebuild the pancreas, it is necessary to wash out the acid accumulation and promote better sugar metabolism. This can be done on a two-day high-mineral fast in which only the broth made of low-starch vegetables that are high in potassium is used.

Potassium Broth: Mix low-starch vegetables, such as celery, string beans, zucchini squash, beets, and parsley, in a blender. Let the mixture simmer, in just enough water to cover it, until it is a broth. Take this *Potassium Broth* throughout the day during your fast. Take no other foods. If you become thirsty between servings, sip some room-temperature water. Take this *Potassium Broth* as your nourishment for two days. You can divide the servings into three "meals" per day if you wish.

Pancreas-Healing Benefits: The potassium can heal and revitalize the cells of the pancreas without interference from other food elements. Furthermore, the low-starch vegetables spare the pancreas of its obligation to release insulin so that the organ can "rest" and "recuperate" while it is being nourished with potassium. The *Potassium Broth* introduces a supply of minerals that help rebuild the islets of Langerhans so that they can release more insulin. Within two days, the pancreas can be rebuilt so that it can function more adequately. The two-day high-mineral fast also neutralizes much of the acidity that is often found in persons with poor insulin production. It is the natural way to heal and revitalize the pancreas.

A DAILY PROGRAM TO PAMPER YOUR PANCREAS FOR BETTER HEALTH

Stimulate your body's circulation through various daily pancreas-pampering programs. Once you stimulate your pancreas, it will function more healthfully and release a sufficient supply of sugar-dissolving insulin. Here are some suggestions for pampering your pancreas:

1. *Warm Shower on Abdomen.* Twice daily, direct a comfortably warm shower on your abdomen for 10 to 15 minutes. Increase the warmth if you can tolerate the heat comfortably. When your skin

turns red, your pancreas has been stimulated by the warm or comfortably hot shower, and it will boost its insulin production.

2. *Eat Yogurt Daily.* As a fermented milk product, yogurt introduces "friendly bacteria" into the digestive system, which stimulates your pancreas for greater efficiency. The yogurt also helps wash accumulated acids and toxins from the pancreas. It creates a cleansing action that enables the pancreas to perform more healthfully.

3. *Eat Raw Vegetables Daily.* Freshly washed and scrubbed raw vegetables should be eaten daily. Select low-starch vegetables so that there is less metabolic effort required of your pancreas. Low-starch vegetables include beets, cabbage, broccoli, celery, Brussels sprouts, Swiss chard, eggplant, lettuce, mushrooms, green and red peppers, and radishes. Raw vegetables also provide roughage to protect your body from toxic accumulation by promoting regularity. You can flavor the vegetables with some vegetable oil, lemon juice, and herbs and spices.

4. *Fresh Air and Exercise for Body.* As often as possible, get out into the fresh air. Take long walks. Get involved in such activities as golf, tennis, swimming, bicycle riding, jogging, and hiking. When you exercise, you send oxygen to all of your organs, and you help stimulate your pancreas so that it can function better.

5. *Eat Only When Relaxed.* Do not overburden your digestive organs and pancreas by eating when you are hurried or tense. You will constrict the muscles and arteries involved in pancreatic health and deprive the pancreas of important nutrition. If you feel "keyed up" or tense before a meal, sit down in an armchair and relax before you eat. Do not eat your meal until you feel contented. Then eat slowly and chew your food thoroughly. Eat well, but do not eat until you feel full. This overburdens your pancreas and leads to improper digestion. Make mealtime a "joytime" as you pamper your pancreas with relaxed eating.

6. *Buttermilk Is a Pancreas-Energizer.* As a fermented milk, buttermilk is a remedial food for the pancreas. Buttermilk appears to regulate the secretion of gastric acid, for it reduces the level of acid. Buttermilk contains lactic acid, which stimulates the pancreas. It helps control blood sugar levels. The lactic acid influences fat metabolism and secretions of the pancreas. It helps stimulate the pancreas so that it can help keep you healthy.

7. *Eat Fresh Tart Fruits Daily.* Your pancreas will be pleased by tart fruits, including tart apples, berries, and citrus fruits, such as

oranges, grapefruits, tangerines, and cranberries. (Drink their juices daily for speedy assimilation by your pancreas to stimulate its insulin production.) You can buy sugar-free bottled, canned, or frozen cranberry juice at health stores or special diet shops. You can make your own this simple way: Cook one pound of cranberries in four cups water until they are soft. Crush them. Drain the mixture through cheesecloth to make it clear. Add a bit of cinnamon powder, vanilla, or honey for flavor. Drink one or two glasses of this cranberry juice daily. Tart fruits and juices have a high alkali content, which increases the alkali reserve in the bloodstream. This helps regulate sugar balance. Tart fruits and their juices can be considered "natural medicines" for healing and invigorating the pancreas.

8. *Use Whole Grain Breads and Cereals.* All breads and cereals should be made with whole grain, unbleached flour. Whole grain breads and cereals contain fiber, which helps prevent sugar overload. On the other hand, refined or bleached breads and cereals contain processed carbohydrates in the form of starch, which is instantly converted into sugar in the digestive tract and bloodstream. This forces the pancreas to release a huge amount of insulin to help metabolize the sugar. The pancreas becomes strained from overwork when the consumption of refined breads and cereals become excessive. The strain causes the pancreas to malfunction. Switch to whole grain breads and cereals. They are converted into digestive starch more slowly so that the pancreas is not overworked.

9. *Use Honey (in Moderation) for a Healthy Sweet.* When you give up refined sugar, you need not deprive yourself of all sweets. You can use honey for a sweet, but use it in moderation because it is a concentrated sweet. Honey appears to be helpful in energizing your pancreas. It is a prime source of potassium, which creates a *hygroscopic power,* the ability to siphon off moisture. Honey tends to draw off moisture in and around the pancreas to help destroy harmful bacteria. Honey is also a prime source of dextrose and levulose (fructose), which are *predigested* sugars. Therefore, honey is easily and gently absorbed into the bloodstream and requires little digestive and pancreatic effort. Unlike refined sugar, it does not put a burden on the pancreas. Use honey for flavoring beverages and whenever you would ordinarily use refined sugar. It is a healthy pancreas-pampering sweet.

10. *Keep Your Body Clean and Your Pores Open.* Take comfortably warm baths or showers regularly. Scrub your skin until it

glows. You should look and feel sparkling clean. The steam from the warm water will open your pores so that toxic wastes can be removed. This helps to clean your entire system, including your pancreas. You will feel your entire body rejoicing with youthful vitality.

Finally, remember to eat an adequate amount of high-protein foods, such as lean meats, fish, dairy, peas, beans, and nuts. When proteins are brought into the intestines, enzymatic action breaks them down into amino acids, which enter the circulation and stimulate the pancreas to release sufficient insulin.

Feel vitality from head to toe with an active and alert pancreas. This organ works with your other body organs to give you a feeling of health and happiness. With proper daily health care, your pancreas can be nourished and invigorated to reward you with energy and vigor.

IN REVIEW

1. To nourish your pancreas, avoid refined sugar in any form.
2. Arlene Q. overcame trembling hands, hypoglycemia, emotional confusion, and excess sugar in her urine with a simple Pancreas-Healing Program.
3. To activate your pancreas, eat sweetbread, whole grain breads and cereals, tart fruits, cold-pressed oils, fish liver oils, and potassium-containing foods.
4. Laurence O' D. helped correct his sugar imbalance with a sweet food. Blueberries and a tea made from blueberry leaves helped boost his pancreas power to correct his problem.
5. Rebuild your pancreas on a two-day high-mineral fast. *Potassium Broth* helps neutralize excess acid often found in persons with weak pancreases.
6. Be good to your pancreas. Pamper it for better health with the ten-step daily program outlined in this chapter.

How to Rejuvenate Your Brain
For Alert Thinking and Emotional Health

14

You can supercharge your brain with youthful energy through a program of healthful foods, inhalation therapy, fun exercises, water applications, and time-tested folk remedies. This program will help boost the youthfulness of your brain, and you will be rewarded with alert thinking and emotional health. Your brain is an organ. Like other organs of your body, it needs to be revitalized so that it can serve you with youthful vitality. Let us look at your brain and then discover the many home methods you can use to boost its energy.

Location of Brain. Situated in the upper portion of the skull, your brain consists of three basic sections: (1) The *cerebrum*, or frontal part, consists of gray matter and associative neurons, or nerve cells. It is believed that this is the site of the intellectual functions. (2) The *cerebellum*, or hind part, is in the lower back portion of the skull. It regulates body balance and helps coordinate muscular movements. (3) The *medulla oblongata*, the lowest part of the brain, is joined to the spinal cord at the base of the skull cavity. It serves as an organ of communication between the spinal cord and brain. It involves such functions as breathing, swallowing, pulse, and heartbeat.

The brain of an adult male weighs about 3 1/2 to 4 pounds. The brain of an adult female weighs a little less, but it is the same size in proportion to her smaller body weight.

The brain contains over 16 billion cells, which require nourishment, oxygen, and exercise in order to serve you well with youthful alertness. Just as you can rejuvenate your other organs through home healing and revitalization programs, you can also boost the youthful vigor of your brain with a variety of home methods.

SWEETEN YOUR BLOOD SUGAR–REJUVENATE YOUR BRAIN

When your brain is given an adequate supply of blood sugar, it can reward you with emotional health, clear thinking, and an alert outlook.

Hypoglycemia: Key to Brain Health. The word "hypoglycemia" means "below normal blood sugar." *Hypo*—below or lower than normal. *Glycemia*—sugar in the bloodstream. It is a blood sugar deficiency, unlike diabetes, which is an excess of blood sugar.

In hypoglycemia, the pancreas has become over-active. It releases too much insulin. This causes body sugar, or *glucose,* to be burned up too rapidly. *The brain cells depend wholly upon blood sugar, or glucose, for nourishment. The brain is usually the first to suffer if there is a blood sugar deficiency as in hypoglycemia.*

THE SUGAR-FREE WAY TO BRAIN REJUVENATION

When you follow a sugar-free diet, you can raise your blood sugar to a healthy level to create a steady supply of nourishing glucose to your 16 billion brain cells.

Avoid Refined Sugar. When you eat food containing refined sugar or refined starch (which is quickly changed into sugar), your body's mechanism for metabolizing this sugar is either triggered too rapidly or is delayed and then set into action too rapidly. In the first case, the blood sugar shows little or no rise following the eating of refined sugar. In the second case, the blood sugar rises, drenches your brain cells to give you quick energy, and then drops abnormally low to give you brain fatigue. This seesaw, up-and-down effect on the blood sugar level leads to erratic emotions. A sugar-free diet is beneficial because it helps stabilize your body's sugar-handling mechanism with slower-metabolizing protein and healthful unsaturated fats. Your brain is then fed a slow but steady supply of glucose so that it can be nourished and reward you with clear thinking and youthful vitality.

Strong Coffee and Tea Upset Brain Health. Coffee and tea are stimulants because of the caffeine they contain. They whip up your adrenal glands and trigger off a glucose reaction similar to that caused by eating sugar. Your brain experiences a quick spurt of energy followed by a sudden drop in energy. You may feel mentally alert and youthful for 30 to 60 minutes as the caffeine whips up your blood sugar, but then you will experience a decline as the effects wear off and the brain is denied glucose. *Note:* Most cola drinks, soda pop beverages, chocolate, and cocoa contain caffeine and create the same "brain fatigue" effect upon your body. Therefore, eliminate these foods from your diet and boost the health and efficiency of your brain.

THE SWEET PROTEIN WAY TO YOUTHFUL BRAIN POWER

Elaine K. R. was often embarrassed by her frequent forgetfulness. In the middle of a conversation, she would forget what she was going to say and even forget much of what she had just said! She would read several pages of a book and forget what she had read. Elaine K. R. was worried. At times her memory was sharp and alert, and then her mind would suddenly go blank! She felt that she was the victim of "brain fatigue." She was afraid of senility. Voicing her fears to a food enthusiast who was also a nutrition researcher, Elaine K. R. asked if there were some natural ways to help correct her faulty memory. The researcher told her that she would have to switch from refined sugars and starches to more healthful sweets and a high-protein diet. Here is the *Sweet Protein Way* that restored Elaine K. R. to youthful health and gave her youthful brain power:

Basic Plan: Follow this program for two weeks. Do *not* cheat since you (and your brain) will pay the penalty.

You Must Avoid:

1. Sugar, candy, cake, pie, pastries, sweet custards, puddings, ice cream, and all other sweets containing refined sugar.
2. Potatoes, rice, grapes, raisins, plums, figs, dates, and bananas.
3. Spaghetti, macaroni, and noodles.
4. Caffeine in any form—coffee, tea, cola drinks, and low-calorie cola drinks.
5. Wine, cocktails, beer, and cordials.

You May Enjoy These Foods in Unlimited Amounts:

1. Asparagus, broccoli, Brussels sprouts, cabbage, cauliflower, carrots, celery, corn, cucumbers, eggplant, lima beans, onions,

peas, radishes, sauerkraut, squash, string beans, turnips, and tomatoes.

2. Apples, apricots, berries, grapefruit, melon, oranges, peaches, pears, pineapple, and tangerines. *Suggestion:* Fruits may be eaten either raw or cooked, but NO sugar may be used. If you buy sugar-packed canned fruit, rinse the fruit twice beneath free-flowing water. Let it stand overnight in water to help remove more of the sugar.

3. Lettuce, mushrooms, and nuts may be eaten as often as you want. *But,* eat only one-half ounce or a handful of nuts at one time.

4. Any unsweetened fruit or vegetable juice, except grape or prune juice, may be taken.

5. Use coffee substitutes such as Postum and herbal teas for beverages. Supermarkets and health stores offer a wide variety of coffee substitutes. You can eat low-calorie gelatin desserts.

Here Is Your Two-Week Plan

This is only a sample plan. Vary the foods to satisfy your taste and appetite. Select items from the preceding lists so that on each day you eat different tasty foods.

On Arising: Medium orange, four ounces of any allowable fruit juice, or half a grapefruit.

Breakfast: Fruit or four ounces of any allowable juice, one egg, one slice of whole grain bread with butter and a beverage.

Two Hours After Breakfast: Four ounces of any allowable juice.

Lunch: Fish, cheese, meat or eggs; salad, a large serving of lettuce, tomato, or apple salad with mayonnaise or French dressing; vegetables if you want, one slice of any whole grain bread or toast; dessert; and a beverage.

Three Hours After Lunch: Four ounces of milk.

Dinner: Soup if you want (not thickened); vegetable; liberal portion of meat, fish or poultry; one slice of whole grain bread; dessert; and a beverage.

Two or Three Hours After Dinner: Four ounces of milk.

Every Two Hours Until Bedtime: Four ounces of milk OR a small handful of nuts.

How Sweet Protein Program Rejuvenates Brain. Elaine K. R. was a "sugar-holic." She was always stuffing herself with sweets, confections, and pastries. She also used sugar to sweeten coffee and tea and drank cup after cup throughout the day. This caused her glucose levels to rise, giving her sudden energy, and then the levels would drop. So she went from alert thinking to confused thinking.

But the Sweet Protein Program offered a slow, steady supply of glucose to the brain so that Elaine K. R. could enjoy restoration of her thinking abilities, giving her the capacity to remember what she was talking about and what she was reading. She was fully recovered from "brain fatigue" after two weeks on this program. She could also satisfy her sweet tooth with the luscious abundance of fruits and juices on this program. A high-protein program had rejuvenated her brain!

HOW SIMPLE INHALATION THERAPY OXYGENATES AND REFRESHES THE BRAIN

With each breath you take, you send a stream of vital oxygen to your brain. When you nourish the 16 billion cells of your brain, you stimulate them into sending forth an electrical charge that is comparable to youthful thinking power.

The Brain-Refreshing Inhalation Program. Select a semi-dark room that is reasonably quiet. Sit on a comfortable chair with your hands on your lap and your eyes partially closed. Stare at a point on the floor about two feet away from you. Take three deep breaths. This helps open channels for the Inhalation Program. Now breathe in and out very deeply and as naturally as possible. *Count your breaths from one to twenty while your partially closed eyes keep staring at the point on the floor.* Count each inhalation as "one" and each exhalation as "two" and so on until you reach twenty. This may sound simple, but it requires emotional and physical concentration.

This *Brain-Refreshing Inhalation Program* takes no more than ten minutes. But it refreshes your brain with a supply of vital oxygen. When you follow this *Brain-Refreshing Inhalation Program* just twice daily, you send *concentrated energy* into your brain cells. In this concentrated form, the air you inhale is like cellular nutrition that helps create concentrated energy, which is especially needed by the *cerebellum,* the brain portion that regulates your body balance and gives you youthful muscle coordination and clear speech. When you follow the *Brain-Refreshing Inhalation Program* just twice daily, you oxygenate and nourish your *cerebellum* and feel rewarded with youthful alertness of body and mind.

FIVE-STEP, FIVE-MINUTE MORNING
BRAIN BOOSTER

Scott F. was afraid of getting behind the wheel of his car in the morning to go to his office. His thoughts were sluggish. His reflexes were dangerously slow. Sometimes he made wrong turns, almost ran into other cars, and averted crashing at the last possible moment. Scott F. always felt "brain tired" in the morning. His responses were dangerously delayed. He had to muster every ounce of brain power to make his hands obey this thoughts. Since he disliked drugs because of side effects, he asked a local physical fitness instructor how he could whip up his sluggish brain. The instructor told of a *Five-Step, Five-Minute Morning Brain Booster* that would supercharge his brain cells with vital energy and give him youthful split-second reflexes. Here is how this inhalation program is followed:

1. Sit erect so that your spine is comfortably firm. At the same time, relax your rib cage so as to avoid pressure on your lungs and other organs in your chest area.

2. Take a long, deep, slow breath and use your diaphragm (muscle sheet between the chest and the stomach) as an air pump. Concentrate upon using your diaphragm to pump air deep into your lungs. At the same time, expand your rib cage, keeping it relaxed and without strain.

3. Now exhale slowly, using your diaphragm to create a reverse action, a squeezing pump that sucks air out of your chest.

4. Continue your rhythmic breathing with emphasis upon your diaphragm as an air pump that takes in the air and then squeezes it out of your system. You should exhale for a little longer than you inhale to sweep out the cobwebs from your brain. That is, if you inhale for five seconds, exhale for seven seconds.

5. Rest for a count of five after each exhalation.

Clears Up Thinking and Rejuvenates Reflexes. This five-step program should be followed for five minutes before breakfast each morning. Scott F. followed the program for one week. Slowly, he found that he could think better and was more alert in the morning. By the end of the week, his reflexes were so rejuvenated that he could drive his car with the hair-trigger reflexes of a teenager!

Benefits of Five-Step, Five-Minute Morning Brain Booster. This regular breathing program improves the oxygenation of the bloodstream, which transports this "air nourishment" to the *cerebrum* portion of the brain, which needs oxygen in order to promote intelligent responses. The oxygen brought by the bloodstream satisfies the "air hunger" of the *medulla oblongata,* which speeds up reflex communications between the spinal cord and the brain. There is a feeling of refreshing rejuvenation of the brain so that thinking is acute, decisions are easy, and reflexes are instantaneous.

This *Brain Booster* is especially helpful in the morning when the brain tissues are "hungry" for air. During sleep, the bloodstream is diverted from the brain so that it may put the body to rest. Nature diverts this blood nourishment so that the brain can be put to healthy sleep. In the morning, the oxygen-hungry brain is sluggish and reflexes are often slow. To help satisfy the brain tissues' "appetite" or "hunger" in the morning, feed them a "breakfast" of healthy oxygen. The *Five-Step, Five-Minute Morning Brain Booster* offers "breakfast" to your brain to energize it like a healthy breakfast energizes your body.

THE BRAIN REJUVENATION SECRET
OF THE TIBETAN LAMAS

The Lamas of Tibet (a mystical and inaccessible land located in the uppermost regions of the Himalayan Mountains between China and India) are known for living well beyond the century mark. Explorers have brought back scientific proof that even though the Lamas (monks) live to be well over 100 years of age, they have thinking abilities that rival those of a youngster. All of the older Lamas could recite tales of their childhood and discuss philosophy, politics, and agriculture with the youthful intellect of a college student. The explorers found that the Lamas has such alert brains that they could even master modern scientific problems with a little bit of training. It took skillful maneuvering for the explorers to discover the basic secrets of the youthfulness of the Lamas. One of the secrets, it is reported, was a simple daily brain rejuvenation exercise practiced by all of the Lamas.

Tibetan Brain Rejuvenation Secret. Assume a posture of meditation. You may sit cross-legged if you are comfortable doing so. Otherwise, sit on a straight-backed wooden chair so that your body is firm, erect, and comfortable. Close your eyes. Breathe in slowly to the count of five. Once you have breathed in for the count of five, hold this breath for another count of five. Then slowly exhale to the count of five. Pause to the count of five. Then breathe in slowly again for the count of five. Repeat this procedure for approximately five minutes.

Important: While you follow this *Tibetan Brain Rejuvenation Secret,* visualize a white circle. Each time you breathe out, make that white circle a little smaller. Continue doing this until the circle is just a pinpoint. Then continue breathing until this pinpoint has become a void. When you have accomplished this respiratory-visual feat, you have tapped the Tibetan secret for keeping the brain young.

Benefits of Tibetan Brain Rejuvenation Secret: When you visually concentrate on the white circle, you insulate your mind and body from outside influences to create a form of brain relaxation and refreshment. When you breathe in the slow rhythm while visualizing the circle, you create a form of cellular cleansing or temporary air relaxation. This washes out accumulated wastes, and for a few seconds you experience a feeling of extreme peace in your mind and body.

As you bring fresh air into your body, your brain is treated to a form of *clean* oxygenation that assures an almost waste-free combustion. This form of oxygenation spares the liver and kidneys. There is less carbon dioxide to be eliminated. The brain receives the full force of this oxygen refueling. The brain, having less toxic wastes, feels its tissues being "swept out" and "cleansed," and it is able to function with more vigor and youthfulness.

In just a few moments, this internal exchange can take place to cleanse the brain, nourish it with pure oxygen, and stimulate the three segments of the brain so that they reward you with youthful thinking. The amazing perpetual youth of the Tibetan Lamas is traced to this *Brain Rejuvenation Secret.* Now you can follow it in your own home for only moments a day. It's absolutely free!

THE ALPHA STATE WAY TO "THINK YOUNG" BRAIN POWER

Brain rejuvenation is traced to the vigor and power of brainwaves. Strengthen the brain waves, and you will enable your brain to function more youthfully so that it can "think young" at any age. This is known as the Alpha State, a condition in which the primary youthful powers of the brain are alerted and activated. When you follow a program that helps you enter the Alpha State, you invigorate your brain. The following program boosts the emissions of Alpha waves, which act as energizers for the brain, giving them rejuvenated abilities.

How to Enter the Alpha State for Brain Rejuvenation

Schedule just ten minutes a day for this program, preferably in the morning when you have your tasks waiting for you and need youthful mind and body strength.

1. Make yourself comfortable. You may sit, stand, or lie down, but you should be comfortable.
2. Look up at the ceiling. Look at a specific object, even if it is only a little crack or a design. Fix your attention on this object. Do not stare, but look at it and relax.
3. Take five comfortable, lung-filling breaths and then exhale slowly. All the while say silently to yourself, "Y...o...u...t...h."
4. When you reach the fifth exhalation, count back to the number one. Now silently say the word, "Alpha." Close your eyes. Keep repeating the word "Alpha" silently as you breathe in and out for two minutes. Visualize yourself as being alert and invigorated at the end of the two minutes, with a strong body and a strong mind.
5. At the end of this *Alpha State Program,* which should take only ten minutes, open your eyes and slowly look around. Soon you will feel vital energy flowing throughout your body. Your thinking will be sharp. Your reflexes will be alert. You will have oxygen-washed your brain, and you will be able to "think young" for the day ahead.

THE HYDRO-HEALING WAY TO BRAIN REJUVENATION

Ordinary water can help cause an internal reaction that makes your brain respond with youthful alertness.

Beth C. C. used a simple *Hydro-Healing Brain Method* to help turn back the hands of time and give her "brain power" that rivalled that of a youngster. Her problem began when she felt her memory faltering. Sometimes she forgot having spoken to people. She frequently forgot appointments. If she marked them down, she forgot to consult her calendar! Simple household tasks confused her. She forgot the names and identities of some of her friends. So it was that a neighbor, a practical nurse, told Beth C. C. that easy water therapy at home could help boost her thinking abilities and rejuvenate her brain. She helped Beth C. C. follow this program since Beth still had a fuzzy memory and might have forgotten the instructions.

Hydro-Healing Brain Method: An oxygen-starved and blood-starved brain suffers cell deterioration, which leads to loss of mental ability. To draw a flow of oxygen- and nutrient-bearing blood to the brain, you need warmth. *Warmth acts as a magnet to attract blood.* Wherever a warming pad is placed, blood flows and deposits healing nutrients and oxygen for deprived cells and tissues. Three times daily, Beth C. C. was given a Turkish towel that had been soaked in comfortably hot water. The towel was wrapped around her throat. The warmth speedily attracted the sluggish blood, which now swept upward and nourished the cells of the upper region, especially the brain. Three times daily this hot-towel treatment helped improve the thinking ability of Beth C. C.

Homemade Thinking Cap. The nurse created a simple but highly effective Homemade Thinking Cap for Beth C. C. She filled a conventional ice bag or a hot water bottle with comfortably hot water. A Turkish towel was put on top of Beth C. C.'s head. Then the bag was placed on top of this towel. The warmth seeped through the towel and stimulated nerve endings in the scalp to draw more blood into the brain. The oxygen-carrying blood flowed upward to nourish, repair, and heal the billions of cells of the brain. This *Homemade Thinking Cap* lived up to its name. It renourished Beth C. C.'s brain and stimulated her thinking abilities. Within seven days, she felt restoration of her "lost mind." Her memory was sharp. Her thoughts were crystal clear. She knew everything and remembered even tiny details. Beth C. C. continues to follow the warm-towel-around-her-throat treatment every day. She also uses the *Homemade Thinking Cap* at least twice weekly. Thanks to this easy Hydro-Healing Program, she feels younger than her granddaughter.

Just as warmth applied to cold hands and feet can stimulate them and restore them to youthful vigor, so warmth applied to the head and around the throat can draw healing blood and vital oxygen to the brain to give it youthful vigor.

BREAKFAST: KEY TO GET-UP-AND-GO
BRAIN POWER

Ted L. habitually raced out of the house without stopping for breakfast. At the factory where he worked as a payroll supervisor, he would grab a cup of coffee and a pastry. Jokingly, he referred to that as his breakfast. But it was no joke when Ted L. started making serious errors in his bookkeeping. Long columns of numbers looked blurred and confusing. Frequently, he forgot to prepare certain statements and schedules. His supervisors called him to task for his incompetence. They said he was "getting old" even though he was in his young middle years.

Only after much questioning did they find that Ted L.'s "senility" or "sluggish brain" was caused by his skipping of breakfast. His problem was made worse because his coffee-and-pastry "breakfast" loaded his bloodstream with caffeine and refined sugar. This played havoc with his blood sugar levels and his emotional health. So it was that a company nutritionist outlined this simple program for Ted L. to follow:

He must *not* leave the house without a substantial breakfast. Each breakfast had to have one or more items selected from the following categories:

Protein Food: Meat, fish, eggs, and cheese. *Benefit:* Protein helps stabilize the blood sugar levels so that they do not fluctuate and can provide a steady supply of brain-feeding glucose.

Healthful Carbohydrate: Any whole grain, unbleached cereal prepared with milk and fresh fruit. He could also eat buckwheat pancakes, millet, oatmeal, unbleached corn products, and whole grain waffles. *Benefit:* Carbohydrates from a whole grain source help complement the protein so that it can be metabolized at a slow and steady rate to nourish the brain for most of the day. They also help provide oxygen to the brain to give it energy.

Energizing Beverage: Milk or a coffee substitute such as Postum or an herbal tea flavored with honey and a slice of lemon. Any citrus fruit juice, because it offers important Vitamin C and minerals that nourish the brain and stimulate it for better vigor. *Benefit:* Nourishes the billions of brain cells.

Vitamins-Minerals. Assorted fresh fruits or a raw vegetable salad with dressing. *Benefit:* The plant nutrients, vitamins and minerals, are needed to stimulate the bloodstream and repair body organs so that energizing oxygen can be transported more completely to your thinking centers.

Ted. L. Bounces Back with Get-Up-and-Go Brain Power. After following this simple program for six days, Ted L. discovered that his thinking capacities were rejuvenated. He could add up long columns of figures without errors. His memory became acute. His attitude was youthful and alert. He was like a youngster. Now he eats his "brain foods" in the morning and is rewarded with get-up-and-go brain power.

Discover a world that is forever young and filled with the joy of living when you supercharge your brain with nourishing foods and oxygen. A rejuvenated brain is a rejuvenated body. Enjoy the best of both worlds by following the home programs outlined in this chapter.

IN A NUTSHELL

1. Sweeten your blood and oxygenate your brain so that it is forever rejuvenated.
2. Switch from refined sugar to the natural sugar in fruit for brain rejuvenation.
3. Elaine K. R. followed a *Sweet Protein Way* for youthful brain power in just two weeks.
4. Try the Brain-Refreshing Inhalation Program for just ten minutes to enjoy more vigorous thinking.
5. Scott F. tried a *Five-Step, Five-Minute Morning Brain Booster* to sharpen his thinking capacities and give him youthful, split-second reflexes.
6. The *Brain Rejuvenation Secret* of the Tibetan Lamas takes only five minutes but may help give you the youthful thinking abilities for which the aged Lamas are known.
7. For "Think Young" brain power, follow the *Alpha State Program.*
8. Beth C. C. overcame her failing memory with a simple *Hydro-Healing Brain Method.*
9. Ted L. discovered youthful get-up-and-go brain power by eating everyday foods for breakfast.

Boost Youthful Energy
Through Adrenal Gland Stimulation

15

You can enjoy youthful vitality throughout the day, feel energy flowing through your bloodstream, and experience clearer thinking, better muscular coordination, and a feeling that the world is a wonderful place in which to live. All this is possible when you have alert and properly stimulated adrenal glands. Youthful energy of body and mind can be your reward for nourishing and revitalizing your adrenal glands. These glands release youth serums, or hormones, that act as "spark plugs" to give you vitality of body and mind. They can give you emotional health and a youthful attitude so that you can deal with stress in everyday living. Healing and revitalization of the adrenal glands can be accomplished through a variety of home programs. But first, let us become familiar with these organs of youthful vitality.

Location of Adrenal Glands. The adrenal glands are a pair of glands shaped something like Brazil nuts. They sit astride each kidney in the small of your back. Each adrenal gland consists of two basic parts, the medulla and the cortex.

Medulla. The inner portion of the adrenal gland, which is an extension of your nervous system. It is your "alarm box" that prepares you to meet the challenges when you encounter stress or danger. When you face physical or emotional danger, your medulla is activated to release a youth serum, or hormone, known as *adrenalin.* A healthy medulla will release this "youth serum" directly into your bloodstream to improve your heartbeat, boost production of vitality-creating glucose in the bloodstream, and strengthen your muscles. In severe situations, the medulla-released "youth serum," adrenalin, may even cause your hair to stand on end!

Cortex. The outer portion of the adrenal gland, which releases *cortisone,* a youth serum that promotes flexibility in the musculo-skeleton system to protect you from arthritis. A healthy cortex that is properly nourished so that it can be activated according to your needs will also guard against rheumatic fever, strengthen the body's connective tissues to protect you from metabolic breakdown, strengthen your resistance to allergies, and give your mind and body a feeling of perpetual rejuvenation. Cortisone will also help regulate your blood sugar levels so that you have vitality and energy through-out the day. It also helps wash away toxins produced by fatigue so that you feel alert and youthful, with a desire to keep active at any age.

Adrenals: Glands of Body Revitalization. When your adrenal glands are supercharged with nutritional energy, your entire body receives the benefits of revitalization. The adrenal glands give you a feeling of youthful energy and vitality. Feed them properly to enjoy natural rejuvenation.

HOW FRUIT ACTIVATED THE ADRENAL GLANDS FOR "TOTAL YOUTH"

As a salesgirl, Louise Du C. should have had a smile for everyone. She had once been cheerful and efficient in the large department store where she worked behind a busy counter. But as time went on, Louise Du C. became temperamental. She was cross. She lost her temper easily. She became quarrelsome with customers. She refused to go into the storeroom to find items that the shoppers requested. Louise Du C. might have lost her job and become a social outcast because of her irritable behavior if a visiting agricultural scientist hadn't noted the problem. He was setting up a special fruit counter, and he heard that Louise Du C., formerly very pleasant, was becom-ing unruly and disagreeable. So he suggested that she follow a simple but effective "adrenal activating" plan. It called for eating a variety of fresh fruits throughout the day. Here is the plan that activated Louise Du C.'s adrenal glands for "total youth":

Adrenal-Activating Plan. Begin each of your three daily meals with an assortment of fresh fruits. End each of the meals with an assortment of citrus fruits. The benefit provided is Vitamin C and minerals, which are needed by the adrenal glands for the manufacture and release of their youth serums. The fresh fruit is metabolized, and its Vitamin C and minerals are transported via the bloodstream to the adrenal glands. These glands then use these nutrients as materials to create their youth serums. These, in turn, are released throughout the body to help protect it from stress and promote a cheerful and bright outlook.

The citrus fruits eaten at the end of the meal are prime sources of enzymes, which metabolize ingested foods and help remove vitamins and minerals that are used by the adrenal glands to create valuable hormones that can change your mood from gloom to cheer and put more vitality into your body.

Feels Happy, Energetic, and Youthful. In just eight days, Louise Du C. had so supercharged her adrenal glands that she now felt happy. She was energetic and walked around the store doing all of her chores with youthful vitality. Her adrenal glands had been nourished and activated through the nutrients in the fruits, and she bounced back with alert vigor. Now Louise Du C. eats fruits daily as the natural way to a happy body and mind through adrenal stimulation.

THE NUTRIENT THAT CREATES THE "JOY OF LIVING" AT ANY AGE

"From Grandma to Glamour Girl in 12 Days." Family and friends loved Rose M. for being a typical grandmother. But even though she was only in her early 60's, she began to show signs of advanced age. Her hands started to tremble. Her skin became parched. When she walked, it was with a slow, stooped gait. Sometimes she needed help to get up from a chair. She felt dizzy when she got out of bed. Noises irritated her. Even the laughs and cries of children annoyed her. She looked very aged. Everyone whispered that she looked as if she were approaching "the end." In brief, the joy of life was gone for her.

A biochemist suggested that Rose M. stimulate her sluggish adrenal glands. He said that she needed one nutrient in concentrated form, along with others, to alert and energize her sluggish adrenal glands. That nutrient was *pantothenic acid.* A little-known member of the vitamin B-complex, pantothenic acid is considered one of the most important sources of food for the adrenal glands. Rose M. was told to boost her intake of *pantothenic acid* by following this easy program.

"Glamour Girl Tonic." Three times daily, drink one glass of this easy-to-make "Glamour Girl Tonic." Into a glass of any fresh fruit juice, stir one teaspoon of brewer's yeast, two teaspoons of black-strap molasses, and one tablespoon of desiccated liver. (These ingredients are available at health stores.) Stir the mixture vigorously. Then drink it slowly. This "Glamour Girl Tonic" is a powerhouse of pantothenic acid, which is needed by the adrenal glands to boost production of their youth serums.

Rose M. followed this tasty program for only 12 days. She began to undergo a total rejuvenation of body and mind. Her hands became steady. Her skin firmed up and took on a "blushing rose" color. She was able to walk, sit, and stand with youthful vigor. She was no longer bothered by noises. She laughed as she said that she had changed from a Grandma to a glamour girl in just 12 days. Now she was ready to taste the "joy of living" even though she was a Grandma, thanks to the "Glamour Girl Tonic."

Benefits: All of the vitamins and minerals work with pantothenic acid in this tonic to nourish the adrenal cortex. The adrenal cortex takes up the pantothenic acid and uses it to nourish its cells to protect it from shrivelling. It also uses pantothenic acid to boost blood circulation throughout the body and wash out decaying cells. Pantothentic acid is the electro-dynamo that sets off production of cortisone and other youth serums needed for total body rejuvenation.

The "Glamour Girl Tonic" (it can be used by males, too!) accelerates the rate of youth serum production by the adrenal glands. It helps boost absorption of nutrients throughout the body. It controls cell and tissue breakdown. It guards against many conditions that cause premature aging. The pantothenic acid in the tonic is stimulated by the Vitamin C and used by the adrenal glands for healthy hormone manufacturing. The entire body is rewarded with energization. It's the tasty way to savor the "joy of living" at any age.

12 WONDER FOODS THAT ENERGIZE YOUR ADRENAL GLANDS TO PROMOTE YOUTHFUL VITALITY

Nutrients in a particular group of foods specifically focus activity upon the adrenal glands. They nourish the adrenal glands and prompt them to release necessary youth serums to protect against age and stress. These "wonder" foods are available in many supermarkets and in health stores.

Basic Plan: Include these "wonder" foods in your regular diet throughout the week. All foods should be as natural and unrefined as possible. Include as many (if not all) of these adrenal-energizing "wonder" foods to help your body bounce back with vigor and youthfulness.

Wonder Food #1—Millet

What Is It? A tiny grain, not much larger than a pin head, resembling a bean.

Adrenal-Energizing Reaction: It contains all ten essential amino acids needed to build and rebuild the structures of the adrenal glands, improving their ability to release youth serums. It is speedily and easily digested. It is alkaline and does not form mucus, so the body organs remain clean and unencumbered. It does not ferment in the digestive system, so your adrenal glands don't have to work too hard to metabolize it.

How to Use It: Use four parts of water to one part millet. Boil the water, add the millet, and reduce the heat to simmer the mixture. Let it cook, covered, until all of the water is absorbed. Add a bit of honey and milk for additional flavor.

Wonder Food #2—Sunflower Seeds

What Is It? The seeds of the sunflower plant.

Adrenal-Energizing Reaction: Sunflower seeds are a prime source of pantothenic acid, which is needed to promote better adrenal action. They provide a good supply of protein to create cells and tissues in the adrenal glands and other organs. They are high in polyunsaturated fatty acids, which lubricate the organs and promote better assimilation of nutrients.

How to Use It: Eat sunflower seeds from the bag, toast them and use them as an appetizer, or mix them with nuts, pumpkin seeds, and raisins for a healthy snack. Add them to cereals, hot or cold. Sprinkle them in waffle and pancake batter before cooking.

Wonder Food #3—Raw Sesame Seeds

What Is It? Small, flat seeds harvested from an East Indian annual herb.

Adrenal-Energizing Reaction: Raw sesame seeds are an excellent source of protein, lecithin, B vitamins, and minerals, which are taken up by the metabolism and used to energize and activate the adrenal glands. They also accelerate the rate of cortisone production and are involved in its utilization by the body so that there is less risk and greater protection against stress.

How to Use It: Sprinkle raw sesame seeds over salads. Add them to any hot cereal. Try cold-pressed sesame seed oil. Munch on the chewy sesame seeds. Roll natural peanut butter, honey, and sesame seeds into little balls for a gland-nourishing confection.

Wonder Food #4—Pumpkin Seeds

What Is It? The ripe seed of the pumpkin plant, usually (and unfortunately) discarded.

Adrenal-Energizing Reaction: Pumpkin seeds provide Vitamin A, phosphorus, iron, and unsaturated fatty acids to nourish the adrenal cells and tissues. They seem to create alertness. That is, when physical or mental stress occurs, the adrenal glands take these nutrients as "fuel" to release shielding hormones that guard the body against cellular breakdown caused by the assault.

How to Use It: Use pumpkin seeds as snacks throughout the day. Add them to cereals and casseroles. Use the seeds with assorted nuts and fruits for a dessert. Pumpkin seeds help give your adrenal glands "pep" after a hard day's work and a heavy meal.

Wonder Food #5—Soy Beans

What Is It? A member of the legume family and one of the best non-meat complete-protein foods.

Adrenal-Energizing Reaction: Soy beans have double the protein normally found in meat. They require less digestive action, so the adrenal glands receive more "purified" protein and more potent amino acids. Soy beans are a prime source of lecithin, a fat-dissolving substance that is needed to "scrub" and "clean" the adrenal glands of debris so that they can work more healthfully. Soy beans are a powerhouse of B-complex vitamins and minerals needed to nourish the adrenal glands.

How to Use It: Soak the beans in water overnight or longer. Cook them in the same water until tender. You may use the cooked soybeans as is or bake or roast them to add to your main meal. They are an excellent meat substitute.

Wonder Food #6—Yogurt

What Is It? A fermented milk product with all the nutrients found in the milk from which it is made. Also known as sour or clabbered milk.

Adrenal-Energizing Reaction: Its fine curd enables its plentiful supply of minerals to be more speedily absorbed for use by the adrenal glands to create "natural tranquilizers" in the system. It helps energize body metabolism, which, in turn, stimulates adrenal secretions of youth serums. Body metabolism is intimately involved with adrenal metabolism, and yogurt promotes adrenal metabolism.

How to Use It: Yogurt is good for eating out of the cup. Mix it with fresh fruit. Add wheat germ, brewer's yeast, or other ready-to-eat grains to it. Yogurt makes a healthy between-meal snack to supercharge an otherwise sluggish adrenal gland.

Wonder Food #7—Brewer's Yeast

What Is It? The dried, pulverized cells of the yeast plant.

Adrenal-Energizing Reaction: Brewer's yeast is the most potent natural source of the B-complex vitamins, which regulate body metabolism so that the adrenal glands release a steady supply of youth serums. Brewer's yeast helps stimulate sluggish adrenal glands through its supply of protein and pantothenic acid and promotes better mental and physical health.

How to Use It: Mix one tablespoon of Brewer's yeast in a glass of fresh juice for a powerhouse of adrenal stimulation in a matter of moments. Sprinkle it over raw and cooked cereals. Add it to yogurt. Use it as a filler or binder in casseroles, meat loaves, and thick soups. Blend a tablespoon of Brewer's yeast with any beverage.

Wonder Food #8—Desiccated Liver

What Is It? The entire liver, selected from healthy cattle, dried and defatted at a temperature low enough to conserve as much of the nutritional value as possible.

Adrenal-Energizing Reaction: Desiccated liver is a good source of linoleic acid, which aids in the transportation of fats, helps the adrenal glands remove excess fats, and then becomes a part of the structural materials found in every cell of all body organs. It is a prime source of concentrated protein, vitamins, and minerals, which become part of the adrenal youth serums.

How to Use It: Desiccated liver is available as a powder, which you can stir into any fruit or vegetable juice to create a powerful adrenal gland energizer. You can also sprinkle it over salads and add it to casseroles, soups, and stews.

Wonder Food #9—Kelp

What Is It? Also known as sea salt, it is made from seaweed.

Adrenal-Energizing Reaction: Kelp is a good source of iodine, which is used by the adrenal glands to nourish other organs, especially the thyroid. The adrenal glands also use minerals in kelp to soothe the nervous system and provide protection against stress. Kelp is a prime source of the potassium needed to stimulate production of adrenal "youth serums."

How to Use It: Kelp is available as a powder for use as a healthful salt substitute. It is also available in tablet form to be taken daily according to the directions on the label.

Wonder Food #10—Peanut Butter

What Is It? Butter made from the seed of the peanut plant, a spreading, leguminous, annual plant. The butter is made by grinding roasted peanuts into a paste.

Adrenal-Energizing Reaction: Peanut butter supplies a highly concentrated plant protein along with most of the B-complex vitamins to help stimulate body organs. The protein is used to nourish the adrenal glands, and the B-complex vitamins are absorbed to become part of the "youth serums."

How to Use It: Use peanut butter as a spread upon whole grain bread with butter or another spread. Use it in a sandwich with lettuce, tomato, and cucumber.

Wonder Food #11—Raw Wheat Germ

What Is It? The seed of the wheat plant, containing almost all of the wheat protein and the oil. Also known as wheat embryo.

Adrenal-Energizing Reaction: This tiny germ is the life of the wheat plant, and it provides the same "life stimulus" to the adrenal glands. Its unsaturated fatty acids help lubricate and clean the adrenal glands so that they can function more efficiently. Wheat germ is rich in vitamins, and minerals, which become part of the youth serums to soothe frazzled nerves and provide better muscle coordination.

How to Use It: Combine it with yogurt for a double-barrelled adrenal-energizing effect. Sprinkle it in cereals, salads, soups, baking, and casseroles.

Wonder Food #12—Fresh Juices

What Is It? A fresh fruit or vegetable juice is obtained by squeezing the plant food with an electric or mechanical juice maker.

Adrenal-Energizing Reaction: Nutrients in the juices are readily available for assimilation by the adrenal glands to provide "instant" energy. That is, within 30 minutes after any juice is taken, its supply of enzymes, vitamins, minerals, and trace elements are working speedily to energize and activate a sluggish adrenal system to release needed youth serums.

How to Use It: Use any assortment of fresh fruits or vegetables to make juice. Enjoy delicious juice any time of the day. You'll experience a natural "lift" and "pick up" with a juice. Its nutrients work speedily. They are attracted to the adrenal glands to be used as "fuel" for making hormones.

In General: Use as many of these Wonder Foods as you want for your meals. You will be building and rebuilding your metabolic system and your adrenal glands will react with youthful vigor as they are stimulated and alerted by these powerful nutrients.

HOW TO SOOTHE YOUR ADRENAL GLANDS IN MINUTES A DAY

Your adrenal glands will react to emotional stress by pumping out more and more hormones to meet the challenges of tension, and they may become overworked. You need to soothe your adrenal glands to prevent them from becoming overworked. You can soothe your adrenal glands in just minutes a day with some simple home programs. Here are some adrenal-soothing programs:

Respiration Soother: You need less than ten minutes for this one. Make yourself comfortable. Be sure that no one will disturb you. Close both eyes. Visualize a lovely scene. It may be the seaside, a cottage in a valley, or a shady forest. Focus your mind's eye upon this lovely scene. Slowly, take a deep breath. Breathe deeply through your nose. Breathe out through your mouth. With each intake of breath, visualize a circle of white energy that envelops your entire body. With each outgoing breath, visualize all tensions, aches, and pains being cast off. Follow this *Respiration Soother* program for ten minutes. It helps soothe and pamper your adrenal glands so that they can *regulate* the amount of "youth serum" being released and not become overworked. Doing this for just ten minutes, twice daily, helps to pamper and soothe your adrenal glands and make you feel good all over.

Positive Thinking Therapy. This adrenal-soother worked effectively for an unhappy architect, Daniel H. K. He was short-tempered. He would get mad upon the slightest provocation. Sometimes he felt exhausted. A co-worker who was an exercise enthusiast told Daniel H. K. that he often used *Positive Thinking Therapy* to soothe his own nervousness. He told Daniel H. K. how to follow this program for just 20 minutes at a time:

Find a quiet place where you won't be disturbed. Assume a relaxed sitting position in a comfortable chair. Close your eyes. Breathe quietly and repeat one of the following phrases: "I am relaxed," "My body will feel younger," or "My adrenal glands are being soothed." It should be a positive phrase that you silently repeat to yourself as you breathe in and out. You will discover that in just 20 minutes your adrenal glands will be more relaxed. They will help control consumption of oxygen, send more blood to your muscles, and build skin resistance so that more body heat is retained. The breathing helps to oxygenate the adrenal glands to create a "sea of air" upon which hormones may then be shipped to your entire system so that you can enjoy freedom from stress and tension.

Daniel H. K. followed this *Positive Thinking Therapy* twice a day, 20 minutes each session, for one week. He emerged feeling healthy, invigorated, strong, and free from his short-temper. He continues to use this *totally free* program at least every other day. He calls it his "adrenal tonic." It has made him feel young and vigorous.

Blink and Breathe Relaxation Program: Sit on the edge of a chair. Place your feet firmly on the floor. Your back should be straight. Your hands should be resting, palms up, on your knees. Gently fix your gaze on a spot before you. It could be a favorite picture, the face of a clock, or a flower in a vase. Once you fix your gaze on the object, do not look away. But you may blink as much as you want to. Take deep breaths through your nose. Then exhale through your mouth. Try not to move any part of your body while you follow this *Blink and Breathe Relaxation Program.* Only your eyelids may move when they blink. Let negative thoughts wash out as you exhale. Become completely passive and receptive to the movement of energy through your adrenal glands. Follow this program for 15 minutes each session. When you finish, you will feel as if your entire body is free from congestions. You will emerge with more youthful vitality.

This *Blink and Breathe Relaxation Program* helps soothe your adrenal glands. Improper eating and unhealthy living tend to whip up the adrenal glands. This overstimulation causes a sudden spurt of "youth serums," which give you needed energy. But the adrenal glands can become overworked and falter, leading to a decline in the production of youth serums. This can cause premature aging. The *Blink and Breathe Relaxation Program* helps soothe the adrenal glands so that they relax. You emerge feeling refreshed and invigorated. In just 15 minutes, you can soothe and pamper your adrenal glands so that your entire body will be rewarded with health and revitalization.

Enter a world of "second youth" by healing and supercharging your adrenal glands with vitality and energy. The adrenal glands hold the key to perpetual youth. Activate, alert, and stimulate your adrenal glands and be rewarded with a "fountain of youth" for your body and mind.

SUMMARY

1. Supercharge your entire body through activation of your adrenal glands.

2. Louise Du C. stimulated her adrenal glands through a fruit program. She became emotionally happy, even-tempered, and a pleasure to work and live with.

3. Rose M. was transformed from the aging Grandma into a glamour girl in just 12 days. She supercharged her adrenal glands with a "Glamour Girl Tonic." It contained a "miracle" ingredient that revitalized her adrenal glands and rejuvenated her from top to bottom.

4. Energize your adrenal glands through any of the 12 delicious "wonder" foods described in this chapter, and be rewarded with youthful vitality.

5. Soothe your frazzled adrenal glands in just minutes a day by following any of the home programs outlined in this chapter.

6. Daniel H. K. boosted his emotional and physical abilities through a *Positive Thinking Therapy* program that pampered, soothed, and regenerated his adrenal glands.

The Five-Cent Food That Helps
Heal and Revitalize Your Colon

16

An everyday food that costs less than five cents per portion has the power to help heal and revitalize your colon and intestines. This simple food is able to offer you natural protection from the problems of cancer of the colon and intestine (the second biggest cancer killer after lung cancer). By using this everyday food, you can build resistance to cancer and heal and revitalize your colon so that it will keep your digestive system working healthfully and youthfully. Your body will respond with energy and vigor.

This everyday food is *bran*. Also known as fiber and roughage, it helps promote regularity and offers protection from cancer of the colon, intestines, and rectum; abdominal polyps of the large bowel; hemorrhoids; and varicose veins. When used regularly, *bran* creates a rhythmical colon action that heals and revitalizes this portion of your body and builds its resistance to many destructive ailments.

To understand what bran can do for your body, let us become better acquainted with your colon and intestinal organs to see how they can be healed, revitalized, and rejuvenated with bran.

Location of Colon. The colon is part of the large intestine. It is a soft elastic tube lined with a thick mucous membrane. It measures about 5 feet long and 2 1/2 inches in diameter.

Function of Colon. As part of the large intestine, your colon has three basic functions: (1) It stores waste accumulation. All food that has not been absorbed passes into the colon. (2) Waste material moves slowly through the colon so that water can be absorbed from it through the colon's wall so that the body won't lose this needed moisture. (3) The colon carries waste material away from the small intestine toward the rectum, where it is cast out.

A healthy colon moves waste materials swiftly so that there is a minimum of transit time. If there are delays, during which these wastes are retained in the colon, a toxic buildup of wastes may cause destruction of colon cells and render them vulnerable to infection and disease. To help maintain a movement of waste materials, eat bran to activate and stimulate your colon so that it will work *swiftly* to eliminate accumulated debris.

A BRAN DEFICIENCY IS A COLON CANCER RISK

A bran deficiency causes prolonged retention of wastes in the colon, which poses a cancer risk. Cancer of the colon is believed to be caused by the growth of bacteria in the stool as it travels through the digestive system. These bacteria decompose bile salts and form new chemicals that are carcinogenic (cancer-causing). Bile salts come from the bile and help digest fats. Once the bile salts finish digesting fats, they are transported through the digestive tract and cast out with waste material.

A bran deficiency causes an unhealthy delay as food travels through the digestive tract. This delay enables bacteria to multiply and create more carcinogens, which also remain in direct contact with the mucosa of the colon, where they may cause cancer, longer. A bran deficiency appears to slow movement of waste materials, and this can cause a breakdown of the colon.

A bran deficiency causes wastes to be smaller so that the carcinogens created by bile decomposition are highly concentrated. These carcinogenic substances in the waste attack the colon, and the cancer risk may become a reality.

Bran: Energizer of Colon. The use of bran daily in the diet will help energize the colon so that it will *speed up the movement of waste materials,* which can then be cast out as quickly as possible. Bran will stimulate a sluggish colon so that it can move vigorously to expel wastes. This exposes the colonic mucosa to very little bacteria contact so that there is a reduced risk of cancer and related ailments.

BRAN—WHAT IS IT?

Here are some of the basic facts about this important food.

BRAN. The outermost layer of the grain seed or kernel; for example, the tough, chewy outer coating of the unrefined wheat kernel. It is separated from the flour or meal by sifting or bolting (a mechanical process that sifts the wheat kernel or grain seed through fine-meshed cloth).

CELLULOSE. A fibrous substance found in the cell walls of plant tissue. It provides bulk by absorbing water as it passes through the digestive system, largely resisting digestion. Sufficient bulk in the bowels helps prevent constipation. (Plant cell walls are complex structures that contain many polysaccharides, such as pectin, hemi-cellulose, cellulose, and lignin. Traces of protein, complex liquids, and inorganic matter are also found in the cell walls.)

FIBER. A substance found in animal and vegetable tissue. Plant fiber is composed of cellulose. *Bran is considered to be one of the best sources of fiber.*

ROUGHAGE. A general term for coarse, bulky food that is high in fiber. By its bulk, it stimulates peristalsis, successive waves of in-voluntary contraction passing along the walls of the intestine to create a bowel movement. Roughage, or fiber, is needed to create regularity to maintain good health.

Bran, whether taken with some liquid or included in baked or cooked goods, is an important food that is needed to boost move-ment of wastes to protect you from "colon congestion," which is often the forerunner of cancer and other ailments. Bran helps create bulky stools, which move along much more quickly so that if any cancer-causing substances are present they have a reduced time in which to be in contact with the walls of the intestines. Bran offers natural protection from colon ailments.

REBUILDS COLON AND INTESTINES ON
25 CENTS-A-DAY BRAN PROGRAM

Troubled with constipation, Vera B. H. was afraid of developing cancer. Somewhat reticent to discuss her problems, she confided to a family friend, a nurse, that members of her family had succumbed to cancer of the colon. She feared that she might be apt to develop the same ailment. She was told that serious or recurring constipation could be a factor in the development of cancer and other health problems. The nurse knew that Vera B. H.'s relations had histories of severe constipation prior to their development of cancer. She under-stood why Vera B. H. was anxious about her problem. So she told Vera B. H. that if she wanted to rebuild her colon and maintain regularity to protect herself from possible cancer of the colon, she should use bran daily.

Simple Program: Each day, take about five tablespoons of bran. (At about five cents per tablespoon, this would come to about twenty-five cents a day.) Vera B. H. used the five tablespoons of bran daily in this simple program: *Breakfast:* Two tablespoons of bran added to any whole grain cereal with milk, added to waffle or pancake batter, or mixed with a fresh fruit juice. *Luncheon:* Sprinkle two tablespoons of bran over any raw fruit or vegetable salad and then add a little vegetable oil, a squeeze of lemon juice, and a bit of apple cider vinegar to complete the dressing. Or add the two tablespoons of bran to a bowl of hot soup. *Dinner:* Add one tablespoon of bran to any casserole, stew, soup, meat or vegetable loaf, or salad dressing.

Regularity Established and Health Revitalized in Seven Days. Vera B. H. followed this program for seven days. Before the week was over, she felt herself becoming regular again. By the end of the week, she was more than just regular, she was more energetic, more revitalized, and more invigorated. The bran had established regularity and helped rebuild the health of her colon. The nurse, a long-time family friend, later confirmed that Vera was free of the threat of colon cancer. Vera B. H. still includes at least five tablespoons of bran daily in her regular diet. It is the tasty and easy way to enjoy regularity and a healthy colon!

THE MIRACLE HEALING POWER OF SIMPLE BRAN

Daily intake of bran can help create a miracle healing power for the colon and related organs. Some of the benefits are:

Creates Internal Regularity. Bran provides bulk that absorbs moisture to create internal regularity without laxatives.

Speeds Removal Time. Bran appears to hasten the removal of waste matter to protect the intestines from exposure to carcinogenic bacteria.

Protects Against Cancer. Bran acts directly on the intestinal microflora, inhibiting or removing the production of cancer-causing substances.

Acts as Insulator. Bran increases the moisture content and bulk of the stool, which reduces the concentration of potential cancer-causing substances. Bran thus blocks their contact with the intestinal wall, creating a "shield" that reduces the risk of colon cancer.

Bran Corrects "Irritable Bowel Syndrome"

Joseph MacB. was troubled by the "irritable bowel syndrome." He suffered from a vicious cycle of constipation, difficult passage of wastes, and diarrhea. Joseph MacB. also suffered from digestive cramps and stomach bloating. (Other names for this problem include irritable colon, adaptive colitis, mucous colitis, spastic colon, and unstable colon.)

Joseph MacB. tried laxatives and cathartics, but they made his problem worse and left him so drained that he felt cold even in warm weather and had the "shakes." His skin was sallow, and his bones were soft. He was taking mineral oil. Like many laxatives, mineral oil tends to absorb Vitamins A and D and wash them right out of the body. This was the cause of his exhaustion, chills, the shakes, and the sallow skin and soft bones. So he wanted a natural program that would ease his colon unrest and boost his general health.

Ten Teaspoons of Bran Daily Correct Lifelong Problem in 12 Days. A co-worker who had the same problem told Joseph MacB. about the easy bran program he followed that eased his "nervous colon." The program calls for taking ten teaspoons of bran every day, to be divided into five "servings." Joseph MacB. took two teaspoons with his breakfast, either mixed with his cereal or mixed with a juice. At about 10 A.M., he added two teaspoons to any fruit juice. He used a spoon to scoop up any residue left on the bottom of the glass, and he would chew this and swallow it. At noon, he added two teaspoons to his beverage or salad dressing. At about 3 P.M., he took a "bran break" by mixing bran in a cup of hot tea or coffee substitute, such as Postum, with a bit of honey for flavoring. At dinnertime, he sprinkled the last two teaspoons into his soup or beverage or added it to whatever main dish was being prepared. This was the simple program he followed daily.

By the twelfth day, Joseph MacB. felt totally "remade." The bran had established normal regularity. His colon had been rebuilt. Gone was this cycle of constipation and diarrhea, and gone were the painful stomach cramps and bloating. Furthermore, he felt warm all over, his hands were steady, his skin looked healthy, and his bones were stronger. Bran *added* health to his colon; the laxatives had *removed* health from his colon.

To maintain the health of his colon, Joseph MacB. feeds it a daily supply of at least five teaspoons of bran taken throughout the day. He is "fit as a fiddle" thanks to his rejuvenated colon.

USE NATURAL WHOLE GRAIN BRAN FOR EFFECTIVE COLON REVITALIZATION

Your colon will be healed and revitalized through the stimulation provided by bran. Since the basic purpose of bran is to cleanse your colon and intestinal tract, the bran itself should be clean. That is, it should be organic, natural, and free from chemical preservatives or irritating additives. When you buy bran, read the label. The label should say that it is "pure," "organic," or "natural" and that it contains no preservatives or additives. Such bran is available in many supermarkets as well as in health food stores. Whole grain bran will effectively create a colon revitalization that will establish regularity and body organ harmony for youthful health.

How Bran Helps Heal the Colon and Intestinal Organs

You may have occasionally chewed raw wheat germ or natural bran. You probably noted the slippery quality that develops when it is chewed. This is a soothing property that heals the colon and intestinal organs.

Bran, as mentioned before, is unchanged by your digestive fluids. It passes through your digestive tract unchanged, and it lubricates and soothes the irritated colon and intestinal walls.

Hygroscopic Healing Benefit. Bran is *hygroscopic,* which means that it retains moisture in the intestinal waste. Through this lubrication, it lessens resistance to the intestinal current. By promoting elimination, the hygroscopic action creates a healing benefit.

Alerts Colon and Intestinal Muscles. Bran contains vitamins and minerals that stimulate the sluggish musculo-nervous mechanism of the colon and intestinal organs. This increases the propulsive force of the movement of intestinal wastes. Bran helps correct resistance to the intestinal current in the colon and intestinal organs. Bran helps improve the propulsive force needed to expel waste. This helps relieve most cases of constipation.

Soothes Spasms. If you are troubled with spastic irritation of the colon, the soothing, bland, demulcent qualities of bran will help relax the spasms and allow a normal movement.

Establish Regularity Without Laxatives. Bran provides your colon and intestinal organs with the roughage that stimulates muscular activity to create regularity. Bran also offers minerals that will both stimulate and support nervous control of those muscles to protect against the constipation-diarrhea cycle and create efficient regularity without laxatives.

Heal and revitalize your colon and intestinal organs and rebuild total body health through rejuvenated organs with the use of bran as a daily food.

HOW TO CORRECT DIVERTICULOSIS
WITH A BRAN PROGRAM

What Is It? Diverticulosis is a condition characterized by the presence of small bulges or "pockets" at weak points in the colon or large intestine. These pouches (diverticula) become packed with wastes and become irritated and inflamed. Sometimes they form abscesses. When food particles and bacteria become lodged in these small sacs, inflammation may result. This causes the condition of diverticulitis.

What Are the Basic Causes? A diet that is deficient in roughage is the basic cause. When your colon is deficient in bran, it becomes weak and cannot function well enough to promote regularity.

It all begins with the colon's need to create peristalsis. These waves of muscular contraction move waste matter through the sacs of the lower intestine. When the bowels are full of this waste matter, the muscles enveloping the intestines contract slightly to move it along.

Roughage creates bulk, which stimulates the colon and promotes peristalsis. If there is a deficiency in roughage, the muscles are forced to contract with greater vigor to create pressure to keep things moving. This is *forced muscular action*. This forced muscular action causes intense contractions in the sigmoid colon (that segment of the colon that leads directly into the rectum), which is lined with strong muscles.

The *forced muscular contraction* causes a buildup of tremendous pressure. The colon cannot cope with such pressure, and repeated pressure may cause the bowel lining to burst through the surrounding muscles to form a balloon, or diverticulum. Over a period of time, many of these diverticula form, especially in the narrow sigmoid colon.

Bran Corrects Weakness. The basic cause of diverticula is *the lack of sufficient roughage in the diet. Bran can correct this weakness. When you follow a high-bran or high-roughage diet, the added bulk allows the sigmoid colon muscles to contract with normal muscular force so that there is little risk of bursting the bowel lining. The key to prevention of diverticulosis is the correction of weakness of the colon through daily intake of bran.*

How Bran Corrected Diverticular Disease

Lisa P. had a history of irritable bowel syndrome. She had severe stomach cramps. She suffered from constipation followed by diarrhea. She was exhausted. Her weak colon was overworked, and the tremendous pressure needed to evacuate it caused "pockets" to form. A neighbor who had the same condition told Lisa P. how she could rebuild the health of her colon and correct her diverticulosis. Here is the program:

Daily, take up to eight tablespoons of unprocessed, natural bran. Mix it with juices or whole grain cereals, add it to salad dressings, or add it to baked goods.

Boost your intake of fresh fruits and vegetables and whole grain breads to provide a greater intake of roughage.

Reduce or eliminate from your diet refined carbohydrates and sugar in all forms.

Symptoms Relieved, Regularity Established, and Pockets "Erased." In two weeks, Lisa P. found that her constipation and diarrhea were relieved. Her stomach pains, nausea, and bloating also went away. Soon she had regular movements with no strain. Later it was found that her diverticular "pockets" were erased. By the end of the third week, her colon and intestinal organs were vigorous and healthy. Lisa P. bounced back with vitality. Now she uses bran all of the time. She radiates youthful health, thanks to a healed and revitalized colon!

A Healthy Colon Means a Health Body. When your colon is healthy, your other body organs can also enjoy good health. It is believed that the carcinogens formed by decomposition of bile salts may be absorbed by the mucosa of the colon and transported to other organs of the body. This may cause cell and tissue breakdown of other organs, and the entire body may succumb. So for good internal health, boost the health of your colon and your other body organs with bran.

From "Stagnant Tank" to "Living River" in Three Weeks

It took just three weeks on a high-bran, high-fiber program for Mark D. G. to transform his colon from a source of accumulated waste to a site of moving health.

Mark D. G. heretofore rarely ate roughage foods. He never ate bran. His diet largely consisted of refined, processed foods. He started feeling bloated, gaseous, and nauseous. Constipation was so common that even harsh laxatives lost their effect. An anatomist told Mark D. G. that his faulty diet was "abusing" his colon and that he needed to invigorate it with high-bran, high-fiber foods. Here is the problem faced by Mark D. G.:

Colon Becomes "Stagnant Pool" With Refined Foods. The colon is the body's disposal plant. It is like a septic tank that holds waste materials between eliminative movements. If the waste cannot be removed speedily, the colon becomes a "stagnant pool." Refined foods that are low or lacking in roughage accumulate in the colon. The absence of roughage weakens the colon and causes *slower transit time.* As a "stagnant pool," the colon becomes infected and colitis may occur.

Colon Becomes "Living River" With Roughage Foods. When the colon is given roughage foods, a natural propulsion is produced and the accumulated wastes are eliminated. Roughage foods cause half-liquid, half-solid wastes to flow through the colon, turning it into a "living river." Roughage creates a "colonic balance" in which solid wastes precede liquid wastes during intestinal movement. This works to keep the colon clean and *reduce the transit time* so that bacterial wastes have less opportunity to become attached to intestinal cells and tissues.

To create this change from "stagnant tank" to "living river," Mark D. G. followed the high-bran, high-fiber program, which worked so effectively that his colon was revitalized within three weeks. Gone was the bloating gas and the feeling of nausea. Regularity became natural, and life became beautiful for the "young" Mark D. G. Here is the simple program that revitalized the colon of Mark D. G.:

Sample Breakfast: Two whole oranges, whole grain oatmeal with bran and milk, whole grain toast, poached egg, and a beverage.

Sample Luncheon: Meat or fish sandwich on whole grain bread; raw salad with a dressing or bran, oil, vinegar, and herbs; whole apple, pear, or raw fruit assortment.

Sample Dinner: Lean meat, poultry, or fish; baked potato with skin; tossed raw salad with dressing and bran; and a beverage.

Snacks: Assorted seeds, nuts, almonds, and sun-dried fruits.

Eliminate: All foods made with refined sugar or starch.

In three weeks, Mark D. G. felt rejuvenated thanks to this tasty program. It rebuilt his colon and other organs and probably saved his life!

14 WAYS TO INCREASE ROUGHAGE INTAKE

Bran remains the basic colon-feeding food. But you can nourish your colon and boost its efficiency through daily intake of other roughage foods. Here are 14 ways:

1. As often as possible, use bran and unprocessed bran cereals with milk or fruit juice. Also use granola, wheat, and oat cereals, dry or hot. Choose the *slow-cooking* cereals rather than the "instant" kind for their higher fiber content.

2. Raw or slightly steamed vegetables offer you a good supply of fiber. A raw vegetable salad topped with yogurt and sprinkled with bran flakes makes a good high-fiber meal-in-a-dish.

3. Use bran for more than a breakfast food. It can be a good dessert. TIP: Combine some natural bran with granola and add fresh fruit slices, a scoop of cottage cheese or yogurt, and some honey. Presto! You have a delicious, natural, high-fiber dessert.

4. Transform soup into a high-fiber food by adding lots of fresh raw vegetables. A scoop of cottage cheese in this type of soup makes a meal in itself.

5. Green pea soup with bran flakes for filler makes a high-fiber food with a gourmet flair.

6. Raw fruits should be your dessert almost daily. Wash fresh fruits and serve them with whole grain crackers for good fiber intake. Add chopped fruits to salads, desserts, and even meat dishes.

7. Citrus fruits are good fiber sources. Peel oranges, grapefruits, and tangerines, *but keep the fibrous membranes* to give yourself good top-notch fiber. Use them for dessert.

8. An assortment of seeds, nuts, and sun-dried fruits make a tasty and crunchy high-fiber snack.

9. On raw fresh salads use natural salad dressings, such as a mixture of apple cider, vinegar, oil, and honey, together with bran. Or you can try cottage cheese, lemon juice, onion or garlic powder, herbs, and bran. A simple dressing is tomato juice spiked with lemon juice, garlic, herbs, and a spoonful of bran.

10. Try a baked or steamed potato. But leave the skin on. (Wash the potato before cooking it, though.) The fiber and most of the nutrients are concentrated in the potato's skin. Keep it low-calorie by moistening it with some hot non-fat milk or cottage cheese and chives.

11. Boost the effectiveness of roughage by using skim milk yogurt. Skim milk yogurt contains beneficial bacteria that alert roughage in the colon to perform more efficiently. Add fresh fruit slices, wheat germ, and bran to the yogurt.

12. With your fiber meals, drink beverages such as fruit and vegetable juices or plain water. The fiber will absorb the liquid and swell up to add needed bulk to your system.

13. Always eat whole grain breads, cereals, crackers, muffins, and so on. These are available in health stores and almost all supermarkets. Read the labels!

14. Try kasha (buckwheat groats), bulgur wheat, couscous, brown rice, unprocessed hominy grits, millet, oats, rye, whole wheat, wheat germ, peanuts, seeds, beans, and peas as other sources of roughage.

Feature a variety of these foods in your meals and help heal, revitalize, and rebuild your colon and the rest of your body.

Bran helps boost the normal action of the colon and intestinal organs during the processes of digestion, absorption, and elimination. This simple food, which costs less than five cents per serving, sweeps your colon clean quickly. It provides protection against infection. It can help rejuvenate your colon and help you look and feel younger, inside and outside, for a long, long lifetime!

IN A NUTSHELL

1. Boost your bran intake to lessen the risk of colon cancer.
2. Vera B. H. eased her constipation problems and fear of cancer with a simple 25¢-a-day bran program.
3. Joseph MacB. ended his "irritable bowel syndrome" problem with a high-fiber program in 12 days. He felt totally "remade."
4. Bran heals the colon and intestinal organs.
5. Correct diverticulosis with an easy-to-follow, tasty bran program.
6. Lisa P. corrected her history of diverticular disease with bran.
7. In three weeks, a high-bran, high-fiber program transformed Mark D. G.'s colon from a "stagnant tank" to a "living river."
8. Rebuild your colon and intestinal organs with the methods presented in this chapter for better total body health.

How Natural Healers Restore
Youth to the Prostate

17

A small organ in the male is his vital link to perpetual youth. This organ determines the effective force and vigor of his maleness. It is strongly related to virility, fertility, and a feeling of "total youth" at almost any age. It is the *prostate*. It is tiny but powerful in its youth-building abilities within the male body and mind. With proper health care, you can heal and revitalize the prostate so that it becomes a gushing fountain of self-perpetuating youth for your entire life. Let us become better acquainted with this "youth organ" and see how it can be stimulated to release important youth serums for virility, fertility, and vitality at any age.

Location of Prostate. Walnut-size and heart-shaped, the prostate is located just below the bladder and seminal vesicles (small pouches in the abdomen just behind the bladder). The prostate encircles the neck of the urethra (the tube through which liquid wastes are carried) as it emerges from the bladder.

Function of Prostate. The prostate releases a youth serum that is part of the seminal fluid that determines the male's fertility. It releases testosterone, the most vital youth serum in the male body. This youth serum is needed by the male for development of sexual characteristics, growth of body hair, and general muscular development. The appearance and feeling of youth are influenced by the quantity and quality of testosterone available to the body. A healthy prostate will release sufficient amounts of this youth serum to help keep the male looking, feeling, and performing with youthful energy.

BODY "WEAR AND TEAR" MAY WEAKEN
THE PROSTATE

Daily "wear and tear" may take its toll on the prostate. Improper nutrition, various deficiencies, and careless living habits cause a general weakening of most body organs. The prostate is often the first to feel the effects of debilitation because it is small, sensitive, and vulnerable. As the body weakens, the effect of "wear and tear" is felt upon the prostate. The male may feel his once-vigorous desires beginning to weaken. He may experience a feeling of premature tiredness. His skin may sag, and his hair may become thin. Overweight may become a problem. These are nature's warning signals that the prostate needs to be healed and revitalized so that the entire male organism can bounce back with youthful vigor and vitality.

A FIVE-STEP PROSTATE-REVITALIZING
PROGRAM FOR SWIFT HEALING

Neil LoQ. was troubled with having to get up at night to make bathroom trips. He was embarrassed by this inconvenience, which annoyed others in the household as well. It interrupted his sleep. He began to look haggard and worn. When he experienced a burning sensation upon voiding and a cloudy urine, he became worried. He sought help from a former classmate of his who was now a professor of urology. The professor told Neil LoQ. that there was still time for him to heal and revitalize his prostate since these were early symptoms. He outlined a five-step program that Neil LoQ. was to follow at once, for seven days. At the end of these seven days, his prostate should be healed and revitalized and the symptoms gone. Neil LoQ. followed the program, and before the seventh day ended, he no longer had to get up at night, he didn't feel any burning sensation, and his urine wasn't cloudy. Here is the easy five-step program that supercharged Neil LoQ. with renewed vitality and energy:

1. *Follow a Raw Vegetable Juice Fast for One Day.* Devote the first day to raw vegetable juices only. Take no other beverages and no other foods. *Prostate-Revitalizing Benefit:* Raw vegetable juices are prime sources of minerals and enzymes that are needed to nourish the prostate. Without interference of other foods, the body can use these nutrients for repair of the prostate and other organs. This helps heal and revitalize the prostate and "repair" it so that it can function more healthfully.

2. *Eliminate Caffeine and Nicotine in All Forms.* These include coffee, commercial tea, cocoa, chocolate, and tobacco in any form. *Prostate-Revitalizing Benefit:* Caffeine and nicotine are "mischief makers" in the prostate gland. They tend to constrict or "choke" the urethra so that there is an obstruction of the flow of urine. This causes a backup and an unhealthy accumulation of waste in the bladder, which may lead to a bacterial infection and irritation in the neighboring bladder. If you eliminate these offenders, your prostate will be able to work more efficiently and pass regular amounts of waste without unnatural storage. Switch to caffeine-free beverages and quit smoking entirely. Your prostate will reward you with more youthful vigor.

3. *Eliminate Harsh Spices and Seasonings.* Omit salt, pepper, ketchup, mustard, and other irritants from your diet. *Prostate-Revitalizing Benefit:* Harsh spices tend to trigger prostate spasms, which cause the prostate to sporadically give off testosterone. There may be spurts of this serum, and then a complete collapse when the effects of these harsh spices wear off. Years of abuse may weaken the prostate and weaken its ability to make testosterone. Use healthful and natural herbs and spices such as paprika, garlic, parsley, oregano, sage, thyme, onion, and others. You will find them in most supermarkets and in health stores. *Caution:* Read labels. Omit any spice or seasoning that contains salt in any form!

4. *Use Vegetable Oils Daily.* Switch from "hard" fats, such as butter or any other animal fat, to free-flowing oils. Use them in cooking and as part of your salad dressings. *Prostate-Revitalizing Benefit:* The tubules of the urethra that connect to the prostate should be kept "clean" and lubricated. Hard animal fats tend to accumulate to "clog" these transport tunnels, which leads to a reduced flow of testosterone. The "clogged" urethral channels also restrict free passage of waste so that accumulated liquids fill the bladder. Men who have to get up nightly will be able to establish regularity through cleansed urethral channels and a healthier prostate by using vegetable oils as a replacement for hard animal fats. You should also switch to low-fat dairy products. Eat more fruits, vegetables, and fat-free products to further protect yourself from prostate "choking."

5. *Eat More Natural, Wholesome, and Unprocessed Foods.* Adjust your diet to include items that are as natural and unprocessed as possible. Eliminate canned, frozen, and pre-cooked foods. A wholesome diet is nourishing to your prostate. *Prostate-Revitalizing Benefit:* Processed foods contain corrosive additives and chemicals

that are injurious to your body organs, especially the sensitive prostate. Since wastes from digested foods pass through the urethra and the prostate, additives and chemicals may burn and weaken these organs and restrict testosterone production. Switch to natural foods, which are more nutritious and healthy for your organs. Fresh fruits and vegetables, lean meats, dried legumes (instead of canned or frozen), whole grains, and fresh fruit and vegetable juices are nourishing to your organs and will boost the supply of youth-building testosterone.

Help heal and revitalize your prostate and other organs with this basic five-step program. It is every bit as tasty as it is rejuvenating.

THE "H-H" PROGRAM FOR PROSTATE REJUVENATION

Nicholas d'A. was embarrassed by his waning vigor. His once healthy male drive was becoming sluggish. When he began to experience difficulty in voiding and experienced vague aches in the region of his groin, he sought out help from a local hydrotherapist. This specialist in healing with water suggested that if Nicholas d'A. had an "enlarged prostate," as all of the symptoms indicated, he needed to follow a 15-minute "H-H" Program for Prostate Rejuvenation; that is, a Hydro-Healing Program that has been used by Europeans for over a century to restore vigor and power to this vital male organ. Here is the program:

"H-H" Program for Prostate Rejuvenation. Fill a tub with *comfortably* hot water to cover the lower part of the body up to the hip line. Sit in this comfortably hot water for about ten minutes, or until you feel warmth and comfort in the region of the prostate. Then draw off the hot water. Fill the tub with *comfortably* cool water to cover the lower part of the body up to the hip line. Sit in this cool water for about five minutes. Then draw it off. Towel dry. Before leaving your bathroom, be sure that you are covered properly to avoid a chill. Keep out of drafts.

Feels Restoration of Vigor and Youth in Eight Days. Nicholas d'A. followed this "H-H" Program for just 15 minutes a day for eight days. At the end of the eight days, he discovered that he felt totally rejuvenated. He was as vital and vigorous as a bridegroom. He had no voiding difficulties. His aches were gone. Nicholas d'A. enjoys a "second youth" at the young age of 54, thanks to his healed and revitalized prostate.

Benefit of "H-H" Program. The hot water relaxes the prostate; the cold water tones up the muscles. The *contrast exercises* the prostate and produces more *rhythmic-flexion* so that its tubules become alerted and are able to release more needed youth-building testosterone. Europeans have used this "sitz bath," as it is called, with much success for more than a century. Now you can follow it in the privacy of your own home. It is absolutely free. It is an effective prostate exercise that can restore vigor to your body and make you feel and act "forever young."

HERBAL HEALERS FOR YOUR PROSTATE

Herbs contain properties that will help heal an enlarged prostate. Herbs will also correct any body imbalance so that there is better elimination and better release of youth serums. Here are some time-tested herbal healers that you can use at home. The herbs are available at most health stores and herbal pharmacies.

How to Cool Burning Prostate. If you experience burning during voiding, prepare the following potion. Mix equal amounts of elder-flowers, buchu leaves, and wild carrot. Use 1/4 of an ounce of each to produce 3/4 of an ounce of the mixture. Add one pint of cold water. Bring the solution to a boil. Turn off the flame. Let the liquid cool. Drink half a cup of the liquid after each meal, three times daily. Nutrients in the herbs will help boost prostate health and soothe and cool the "burning" sensation that accompanies voiding.

Watermelon Seed Tea. Boil three tablespoons of watermelon seeds in one pint of water. Strain the mixture and let it cool. Take one tablespoon of this tea every hour until you feel relief from any discomfort of the prostate.

Ginseng for Prostate Youth. This Korean herb (available in most health stores and herbal pharmacies) has been used to rejuvenate the prostate for nearly five thousand years! While ancients may not have been able to identify or describe the prostate, they knew that ginseng tea promoted rejuvenation—it acted as a youth tonic. Ginseng contains beneficial tonic and revitalizing properties. It has a stimulating effect upon the prostate. It helps restore and maintain the healthful functioning of the prostate. Use ginseng tea regularly.

HOW TO MASSAGE AND ALERT
A SLUGGISH PROSTATE

Years of improper care may weaken the prostate and make it sluggish, resulting in such symptoms as pains in the lower back, constipation, difficulty in urination, and disturbed sleep because of a desire for frequent nightly voiding. Many males feel a sluggish prostate in "lost youth," a loss of virility. Just as any organ becomes inefficient through lack of exercise or massage, so the prostate can become sluggish. You can massage and invigorate your prostate in this simple manner:

When to Perform: Fifteen minutes in the morning and then fifteen minutes at night. Do it for 14 days, and you will soon feel total revitalization through alerting of the prostate.

How to Perform: Lie down on your back, preferably on a hard surface such as a bench or floor. Draw your knees up to your chest, *making sure that your knees and ankles are kept together.* (If you open your knees when pulling them up toward your chest, the exercise is less effective.) When your knees and ankles are as high as is comfortably possible, slowly open your knees and bring your soles together. Now kick your legs out straight so that your heels are two or three feet above the floor. Let your feet drop to the floor. Repeat this procedure ten times, morning and evening.

Benefit: Gentle pressure is brought to bear upon the pelvic area, which houses the prostate. This rhythmic pressure has a massaging and exercising affect upon the prostate so that stored wastes are released and a free waste flow is permitted. It also alerts the prostate and stimulates this organ to release more needed testosterone, the youth serum that helps promote the desire and vigor of youth in males of all ages!

THE MAGIC MINERAL THAT ENERGIZES
THE PROSTATE

Zinc is a magic mineral in that it reportedly is able to energize the prostate and supercharge the body with vitality and youthful vigor. The prostate is known as the "zinc center" of the male body because it needs this mineral more than any other nutrient. Zinc is absorbed by the prostate and is a major component of testosterone, the youth serum.

It has been discovered that men with prostate trouble also show low levels of zinc in that organ. Zinc can help energize the prostate in the following ways:

1. Zinc is able to restore vigor and reduce low back pain, a symptom of prostate weakness.

2. Zinc energizes the prostate to keep the urethral canal clean and protect it from waste formation, which is noted through painful voiding.

3. Zinc boosts the effectiveness of the bladder and intestines so there is freedom from constipation and the sense of unrelieved fullness in the bowels.

4. Zinc also helps maintain a normal control over voiding so there is less difficulty in starting or stopping the stream.

Zinc Corrects Prostatic Disorders. In a reported situation,[1] Irving M. Bush, M.D., of the Center for the Study of Prostatic Diseases at Cook County Hospital in Chicago, Illinois, stated that men who had prostate trouble were diagnosed as being very low in zinc. Dr. Bush gave prostate-troubled men zinc supplements in the amounts of 50 to 150 milligrams per day for two to sixteen weeks. He reports that seven out of ten patients were relieved of symptoms ranging from painful voiding to loss of vigor. Most of the men suffered from benign prostatic hypertrophy (enlargement of this organ), but after taking the prescribed 50 to 150 milligrams of zinc per day over a period of four months, they experienced much shrinkage of the prostate. Zinc supplements are available at all pharmacies and health stores.

Food Sources of Zinc. This prostate-alerting mineral is found in wholesome and unrefined foods such as whole grains, fresh fruit, green leafy vegetables, and organ meats.

Tasty Liver Tonic: Into a glass of tomato juice, stir one tablespoon of desiccated liver powder (available at health stores). You can flavor it with a bit of lemon or lime juice. Stir the mixture vigorously. Drink three glasses of this *Tasty Liver Tonic* daily. It is a prime source of zinc, the mineral that nourishes your prostate and

---

[1] Press release issued August, 1975.

then enters into the prostate fluids such as testosterone to promote youthful vigor and vitality.

THE PROSTATE-ENERGIZING FOOD
FROM THE BEEHIVE

A food that is directly involved in reproduction can help energize the prostate so that it will maintain its powers of fertility. That food is *bee pollen.*

What Is Bee Pollen? Bee pollen is the male sex cells of flowering plants. It is used as food by the bees. It is a very fine powder that is gathered by bees in microscopic amounts and brought to the hive for food. In the process of collecting and depositing the pollen in the hive, bees treat the pollen by adding a small amount of nectar to it, forming it into tiny granules to make it manageable. Many of these granules fall to the floor of the hive, where beekeepers sweep it up, and then it is prepared into tablet form for easy use. Bee pollen is a powerhouse of zinc, the mineral that energizes the prostate and is a large component in the prostate "youth serum" testosterone.

What Does Bee Pollen Contain? A large amount of lecithin, a fat-dissolving substance that helps keep the arteries and tubules of the prostate clean of accumulations. It also contains almost all of the amino acids that are needed to boost the health of the prostate so that it can function youthfully. It contains almost all of the 22 elements of which the human body is composed.

How Will Bee Pollen Energize the Prostate? Bee pollen contains all of the nutrients needed to nourish and energize the prostate. It relieves prostate infection and hypertrophy because it is rich in essential fatty acids, enzymes, zinc, and other minerals that nourish the prostate. It has an anti-bacterial effect, which means that there is a reduced incidence and severity of infection and enlargement. Bee pollen helps prevent leukocytosis (abnormal increase of white cells) in the prostate and cleanse the organ of infectious organisms. It tends to strengthen the prostate so that it can youthfully protect itself against infection.

Pollen is also rich in *testosterone, epitestosterone,* and *androstenedione.* These are three youth serums released by the prostate. When bee pollen introduces these youth serums into the system, the prostate gland takes them as "energizers" and uses them in the manufacture of its own testosterone. Bee pollen is natural food for the prostate gland.

Where Is Bee Pollen Available? Bee pollen is available at most pharmacies and health stores in convenient tablet form.

How Much Bee Pollen Should Be Taken Daily? Reportedly, 500 milligrams daily will offer your prostate the nourishment it needs to release important "youth serums" to help protect against disorders and promote vitality and vigor at any age.

Tap the hidden wellsprings of perpetual youth by improving your prostate. It will function vigorously and reward you with extended youth, vitality, and health for your body and mind.

SUMMARY

1. Neil LoQ. used a five-step program to help heal his prostate and enjoy more youthful vigor and vitality.

2. A simple and free "H-H" Program rejuvenated Nicholas d'A. as he overcame prostate trouble.

3. Herbs are prime sources of concentrated ingredients that will help heal and rejuvenate your prostate.

4. Energize a sluggish prostate with zinc, a "magic mineral" that can help revitalize your entire body.

5. A *Tasty Liver Tonic* is a prime source of prostate-energizing zinc.

6. Bee pollen, a food prepared by bees, reportedly is a power-house of substances that heal, revitalize, and rejuvenate the prostate and the entire body.

"Forever Female"
Through Organ-Revitalization

18

Stimulate the release of youth serums from a pair of organs in the body and you can become "forever female."

To enjoy the look and feel of youthful health, women can heal and revitalize these organs so that they release a steady supply of these all-important youth serums.

Located within your body is a pair of organs known as the *ovaries.* During a woman's fertile years, these organs release hormones that help regulate the monthly cycle of ovulation and menstruation. These hormones, or youth serums, also determine a woman's fertility, enter into harmony with other organs, and help give her firm skin, a youthful appearance, and characteristic feminine curves. During the middle years, the ovaries may become sluggish and release fewer "youth serums." This may lead to a decline in feminity and general health. To help maintain and extend the prime of life, it is important to heal and revitalize the ovaries so that they can continue releasing their all-important "youth serums." This can be done through various home programs. Let us become acquainted with these important organs and see how to use home programs for their healing and revitalization and become "forever female" through your alerted youth serums.

Location of Ovaries. The ovaries are two small organs, each about the size and shape of an almond, set in the pelvic cavity just below the navel. One is about three inches to the right and the other about three inches to the left of the middle of the body.

Function of Ovaries. In a woman's fertile years, the ovaries produce ova (human eggs), which unite with sperm. The ovaries perform another vital function. They work together with the pituitary gland to release *estrogen,* a youth serum that keeps women looking and feeling feminine, gives her skin a youthful texture, and helps give her the glow of youth. A healthy pair of ovaries will continue releasing *estrogen* for most of a woman's life so that she will continue to be "forever female" in body and mind. It is important to keep the ovaries healthy and alert so that they can continue cooperating with the equally healthy and alert pituitary gland to release a steady supply of *estrogen,* the vital "youth serum."

HOW A MINERAL TONIC BOOSTED REJUVENATION

Edith X. was in her middle 40's, but she looked as if she were in her late 60's. Her hair was frizzy. Her skin was wrinkled. She walked with a stooped gait. She had a "coarse" appearance. She was so irritable that she would snap at the slightest provocation. She alienated her family and friends because of her "distemper," as her husband called it. Edith X. had always been pleasant. But when she approached her middle years, she neglected herself. She had taken her youthful health too much for granted. She began to treat her health carelessly. She started taking refined foods, pastries, and sugary beverages. Her vital organs became "starved" and started to react. She was so jittery and irritable that she could hardly hold a cup in her hand without trembling or slamming it down on the counter. She lamented that she was getting old, and she felt bitter about it.

A sympathetic friend who was married to an endocrinologist told Edith X. that she needed to alert and stimulate her sluggish ovaries. She explained that in the middle years these organs may become slow in their production of "youth serums" and need to be alerted and awakened through proper mineralization. She advised Edith X. to try a special Mineral Tonic that her husband often recommended as a way of healing, revitalizing, and alerting sluggish ovaries. Edith X. prepared it according to the simple instructions.

Mineral Tonic for Rejuvenation. To one glass of skim milk, add one teaspoon of brewer's yeast powder, one teaspoon of honey or blackstrap molasses, and one teaspoon of bran or wheat germ. Stir the mixture vigorously and then drink it slowly. Take one glass of the tonic in the morning, another glass at noon, and a third glass at bedtime.

How Mineral Tonic Rejuvenates Organs. The calcium in the milk combines with the B-complex vitamins in the brewer's yeast. Together, they unite with Vitamins A and D in the other ingredients to trigger the pituitary to prod the sluggish ovaries into secreting *estrogen*, the youth serum that keeps a woman "forever female." The calcium is especially important since middle years call for boosted intake of this mineral. There is a greater demand on the organs that need calcium. A calcium deficiency may cause nervous disorders and bone fragility, which results in sagging skin and stooped posture.

Looks Younger and Feels Alert in Eight Days. Edith X. took this Mineral Tonic three times daily, eliminated sugar and salt in all forms, and ate wholesome and unprocessed foods to create a miracle of rejuvenation. Within eight days, Edith X. became pleasant in disposition and attitude. Her hair was shiny. Her skin was firm and showed no wrinkles. She walked with the "bounce" of youth. Gone was her "distemper." In its place was the cheerful disposition of a young and happy woman. All of this was accomplished in eight days. Edith X. still takes her Mineral Tonic three times daily and enjoys youthful health from within and without.

HOW TO "OIL" THE OVARIES AND EXTEND THE LIFELINE OF YOUTH

Free-flowing, polyunsaturated oils are prime sources of essential fatty acids and Vitamin E, which are highly valuable organ-healing and organ-revitalizing elements.

EFA and Vitamin E Helped Extend Youth Lifeline. During the middle years, the ovaries tend to reduce their production of ova. This signals the end of the ability to reproduce. With the end of the fertile cycle, the cells and tissues of the ovaries may wither and become dehydrated because there is less *estrogen* being released. At this time, there is a special need for a pair of important "stimulants" to alert the sluggish ovaries so that they can continue to release needed *estrogen*. These two "stimulants" work in harmony. They are:

Essential Fatty Acids: Essential fatty acids guard against the accumulation of cells and tissues that clog the ovaries and block the flow of needed youth serums. They also tend to dissolve fat particles, which inhibit circulation and block nutrients that the ovaries need. Essential fatty acids, EFA, help cleanse the cells and tissues to promote a better transfer of nutrients from the bloodstream to the ovaries. They help initiate a free flow of essential youth serums.

Vitamin E: Vitamin E helps increase the supply of oxygen so that the ovaries are not denied needed "air." Vitamin E will help dilate or expand the narrow arteries and tubules leading to and from the ovaries so that important nourishment and oxygen can reach these organs. Vitamin E protects the ovaries from *anoxia* (lack of oxygen), which could otherwise cause these organs to dry up, shrivel, and age. Vitamin E nourishes the ovaries so that they can continue releasing needed youth serums to keep you looking, feeling, and acting "forever young."

Garden of Eden Formula. Stella O' B. began to look old. As a dress designer, she needed to look as bright and colorful as her fashions. She feared losing clients. Some people suggested that she needed a vacation. Others said that she looked tired. But one client told her that she had been given an easy-to-follow formula by a visiting internist that was created to rejuvenate and activate sluggish ovaries. The client told Stella O' B. that many women in the middle years need to stimulate their ovaries so that they can remain "forever female" no matter what the calendar said. The simple formula worked for the client, who admitted to being "over 60" but looked under 30. This program gave Stella O' B. an extended lifeline and a return of youthful vigor and energy. She prepared the following:

Into a glass of any citrus juice (orange, grapefruit, or tangerine), she stirred two tablespoons of peanut oil, two tablespoons of safflower seed oil, and two tablespoons of wheat germ oil. She added a pinch of cinnamon or honey for flavoring. She stirred the mixture vigorously. She drank one glass of the mixture in the morning, another at noon, and a third in the evening.

Benefits of Garden of Eden Formula: The free-flowing, polyunsaturated oils in this formula are powerhouses of essential fatty acids and Vitamin E. These are taken up by the Vitamin C of the citrus juice, which acts as an energizer to boost assimilation of the nutrients. The Vitamin C actually "shoots" or "propels" the EFA and Vitamin E through the bloodstream to the ovaries, where they work to alert, activate, and amplify the release of vital *estrogen* and other youth serums needed for "perpetual youth."

Within six days Stella O' B. felt renewed vigor. She had roses in her cheeks. She bubbled over with youthful enthusiasm. She was more successful than ever as an energetic dress designer, and she said "goodbye" to her calendar age of "over 50." She now felt like 20 and looked it, too!

Suggestions: Feed your ovaries and other organs a daily supply of essential fatty acids and Vitamin E by using free-flowing, polyunsaturated oils daily. Use these oils as a replacement for fat. Use oils instead of butter or margarine. Use oils for cooking. Combine oils with apple cider vinegar or a citrus juice to make a salad dressing. Use different combinations of oils with a citrus juice for refreshing cocktails. A variety of oil is available at any supermarket and many health stores. You can enjoy safflower seed oil, soybean oil, wheat germ oil, avocado oil, almond oil, corn oil, linseed oil, peanut oil, rice oil, sesame seed oil, walnut oil, and olive oil. Use them regularly to boost your ovaries so that you can enjoy being "forever female."

AN OVARY-REJUVENATION PROGRAM FOR THE FEELING OF TOTAL YOUTH

Stimulate your ovaries so that they will release rejuvenating hormones to help keep you looking and feeling young. Here is a daily program that is easy to follow and highly rewarding:

1. *Avoid Temperature Shocks.* Do not subject your ovaries to sudden temperature shocks. That is, don't go from a hot house to a cold street or a very cold room into the hot outdoors. Such temperature shocks can play havoc with your ovaries, produce chills, and interfere with a healthy hormone flow. Gradually adjust to different temperatures.

2. *Bathe in Warm Water.* Treat yourself regularly to a leisurely warm bath. You may add epsom salts (one cup to an average tub). A warm bath helps soothe your body and pamper your ovaries with a feeling of warmth and contentment.

3. *Keep Hands and Feet Warm.* Warmth should be equally distributed throughout your body. Keep your hands and feet warm with woolen gloves and warm hosiery or socks. This will protect you from a blood shortage in your extremities and accumulation in other body parts. If your hands or feet are very cold or numb, soak them in comfortably hot water until you feel the warmth returning to your limbs.

4. *Select Wholesome, Natural Foods.* These include fresh fruits, vegetables, whole grains, lean meats, skim milk dairy products, seeds,

and nuts. Avoid processed, refined, bleached products that contain additives and preservatives. Your body organs, such as your ovaries, need the nutrients found in wholesome foods. They will react negatively if they are abused with the chemicals found in refined foods.

5. *Eliminate Salt and Sugar From Diet.* Salt absorbs water and may cause an unnecessary weight gain in the middle years. Your ovaries can become overburdened with this excess weight and will not function properly. Sugar adds calories and also destroys B-complex vitamins. Your ovaries will "protest" by becoming irritable and nervous. Replace salt and sugar with herbs and spices, honey, maple syrup, and molasses to satisfy your taste buds.

6. *Boost Calcium Intake.* During the middle years, a sluggish ovary may lead to nervous irritability. The ovaries need calcium, which they use to manufacture *estrogen* and other youth serums. The ovaries will also use calcium to soothe the nervous system as more "youth serums" are created. Feed this essential mineral daily to your ovaries. Calcium is found in skim milk dairy products; greens, such as turnips, collards, kale, and mustard greens; broccoli, salmon, and cabbage. Eat these foods daily to boost your calcium intake and nourish your ovaries.

7. *Exercise Your Ovaries.* Stimulate the release of more youth serums through a simple "ovary exercise." Here's how: Sit on the floor (on a blanket or towel to avoid being chilled) with your feet extended in front of you. Raise your arms to the ceiling, locking your thumbs together. Breathe deeply, in and out. Stretch your arms out over your legs until you reach your toes. Take hold of your toes and let your head hang loosely. Relax your shoulders. Breathe deeply and casually, focusing your breath on your lower abdomen. Stretch and finish by putting hands on your lap. Repeat this exercise up to six times daily. This "ovary exercise" takes only three minutes, but it will help boost the release of important youth serums.

8. *Twice-Weekly Epsom Salt Bath.* A sluggish pair of ovaries will often result in water-logged tissues. This condition is known as edema. This problem faced Dorothy E. R. At the age of 57, she was pudgy in face and body. She needed to dispose of the accumulated water. She had to stimulate her ovaries to get rid of the excess water. A hydrotherapist told her to use a simple epsom salt bath twice weekly. Dorothy E. R. soaked in the bath every Monday and Wednesday. Within three weeks, the water had been "washed out" of her system and she was slim in face and body. *How to Take the Bath:* Toss one cup of epsom salts (also known as magnesium sulfate)

into a tub of comfortably hot water. Swirl them around with your hand until they are dissolved. Climb in and soak yourself for about 30 minutes. The water temperature should be about 100°F. When you begin to perspire freely, climb out, dry off, wrap yourself in a warm robe, and cool off gradually. *Organ-Healing Benefit:* The heat of the water will open your pores. The epsom salt vapors enter your pores and alert your body organs, especially your ovaries. The vapors cause your organs to eliminate uric acid and help restore blood alkalinity by drawing out accumulated salts. The vapors "dissolve" salt accumulations in the ovaries. The opened pores then discharge the accumulations, toxins, and wastes. Once cleansed, the ovaries can function more efficiently in releasing needed youth serums to prolong the prime of life.

9. *Alert Ovaries With Simple Vibrations.* Wake up your sleeping ovaries with vibrations. Place one hand on your lower stomach just below your navel. Place your second hand on top of your first hand. Move your hands up and down gently. This exercise sends vibrations through your stomach and into your ovaries. It alerts your ovaries. Move your hands up and down ten times. Then relax. Repeat at least twice daily. This exercise helps alert your ovaries and improve their powers of creating youth serums for better health.

10. *Wear Comfortably Fitting but Not Tight Garments.* Your organs can function healthfully only when they are not restricted, bound, or "imprisoned" in any way. Clothes should be comfortable but not tight. Avoid tight undergarments, elastic bands, belts, and footwear. They tend to "choke" the bloodstream and make your ovaries undernourished. In particular, all bedwear should be comfortable and loose so that your bloodstream can nourish your ovaries while you sleep. You will awaken more youthful and healthy through this simple "organ freedom" program.

Heal and revitalize your ovaries through this easy-to-follow ten-step program. It is your key to perpetual youth!

Nutritional Guidelines for Ovarian Health. Your diet should include protein to nourish your ovaries and build their health. You also need Vitamin A to keep the ovarian membranes in youthful condition. You need B-complex vitamins to guard against stress when the ovaries are weak. You need Vitamin C to create collagen, the substance that heals the cells and tissues of the ovaries. You also need Vitamin D to aid in the absorption and utilization of calcium to build healthier and more alert ovaries and, hence, more youth serums. You also need Vitamin E to boost your metabolic processes and to help prevent the formation of toxic substances in your ovaries. You need all of these minerals and vitamins for your ovaries to maintain a healthy water balance and to create a soothing effect.

You can obtain these nutrients from a wholesome, natural diet that includes lean meats, fish, skim milk dairy products, whole grains, lots of fresh fruits and vegetables, fresh juices, seeds, nuts, and beans. A wide variety of these foods are available at supermarkets and many health stores. With these foods, you can actually feast your way to youth through organ nourishment. Your ovaries and other body organs will work in harmony to create a feeling of being "forever youthful" and "forever healthy" thanks to the release of youth serums.

Become "forever female" through ovary revitalization. Your entire body and mind will respond with the radiance of the joy of youth!

IN REVIEW

1. Edith X. turned back the hands of time and became youthful again by taking a *Mineral Tonic* to boost the rejuvenation powers of her ovaries.

2. Essential fatty acids and Vitamin E can help extend your youth lifeline.

3. Stella O'B. took a *Garden of Eden Formula* to stimulate her sluggish ovaries. In six days, she bounced back to youthful vitality and appearance.

4. Follow the easy ten-step program that rejuvenates your ovaries and gives you the feeling of total youth.

5. Dorothy E. R. takes a twice-weekly epsom salt bath. This helps her ovaries wash out accumulated salt and water. She went from "pudgy" to "slim" in just three weeks.

6. Nourish your body by following the nutritional guidelines in this chapter, and boost the power of your ovaries to release an abundance of youth serums.

How to Revitalize Your Thyroid
For Super Energy and Youthful Slimness

19

Supercharge your body with super energy and shed unwanted pounds and inches through revitalization of your thyroid. This small organ can help boost your metabolism so that nutrients work more effectively to give you a feeling of vitality and energy. This organ determines the rate at which your body consumes food and the amount that will be stored or metabolized, thereby controlling your weight.

When you heal and revitalize your thyroid, you can regulate its activities so that you can then enjoy pep, vitality, and youthful slimness. Let's take the mystery out of this organ and see how you can use everyday foods and simple programs to boost its health-giving powers.

Location of Thyroid. Shaped like a butterfly, the thyroid is an endocrine gland that rests against the front of the windpipe. It consists of two lobes, one at either side of the Adam's apple, joined at their lower ends by a bridge of tissue across the upper part of the trachea (windpipe).

Function of Thyroid. It releases thyroxine, a youth serum that determines body growth, regulates the burning of food in your body, influences emotions and personality, and regulates your weight. Too much thyroxine (hyperthyroidism) speeds up metabolism and may cause goiter, an enlargement of the thyroid. Too little thyroxine (hypothyroidism) causes skin distress, puffy face and hands, and low body temperature. A healthy balance is possible through iodine-nourishment of this organ and an adequate supply of protein.

HOW IODINE CREATED SUPER ENERGY
THROUGH THYROID REGULATION

Earl McC. felt listless and indifferent to his work as a construction supervisor. At times he could hardly keep his eyes open by midday. When he was found sleeping in a storeroom in the early afternoon, his superior told him to either stay awake and do his job or he would be fired. Earl McC. was so sluggish that he could not even complain that he was not in control of his functions. He was becoming a robot! His symptoms were noted by a co-worker, who said that his wife had experienced the same "blahs" and had been on the verge of collapse from fatigue when her physician put her on an iodine-boosting program that nourished her thyroid so that it could release balanced amounts of thyroxine, the youth serum that created super energy.

Becomes Energetic and Youthfully Alert in Four Days. The program was outlined for Earl McC., who followed it immediately since he was threatened with job and health loss. Here is the program:

Seafood Daily. For lunch and dinner, Earl McC. ate seafood, which is a prime source of iodine, the mineral that activates and revitalizes the thyroid so that it can release its energy-boosting thyroxine. He ate salmon, haddock, cod, sardines, tuna, or any other deep-water, salt-water fish.

Iodine-High Vegetables. Green, leafy vegetables, brown rice, watercress, and onions, were part of his salad every single day.

Sea Salt Daily. As seasoning, Earl McC. used sea salt or kelp. Sea salt is a powerhouse of iodine. It is seaweed that is dried, pulverized, and made in the form of a powder. It contains all of the rich minerals from the ocean depths, especially iodine. It is available at all health stores and many supermarkets. Sprinkle it on foods as a healthy thyroid-regulating salt substitute.

Bounces Back With Vigor. Almost immediately, Earl McC. could feel his thyroid becoming revitalized. He felt warmth throughout his body. He was alert and active. His mind was bright. He no longer felt groggy. He even looked forward to working overtime. Within four days, he had bounced back with youthful vigor, thanks to this simple thyroid-revitalization program.

How Iodine Can Help Give You a Youthfully Slim Shape

Iodine, a mineral found in foods that are grown close to the ocean or taken from the ocean, can help regulate your thyroid and take off unwanted pounds. With proper iodine nourishment, your thyroid can give you a youthfully slim shape.

When you eat iodine-containing foods, your body stores much of it in your thyroid. A mechanism controls the release of thyroxine into your system. It sends a steady supply of this youth serum, which burns up calories and helps take off unwanted pounds and inches.

Thyroxine, which contains iodine, accelerates the release of energy in the tissues through combustion of glucose. With a stepped-up rate of combustion, overweight can be controlled. Pounds and inches can be melted through the action of the iodine-nourished thyroid.

An iodine deficiency will slow up the function of the thyroid and reduce its flow of thyroxine. This may lead to added pounds and inches.

Your thyroid must have adequate amounts of iodine. Even a slight deficiency may mean the difference between youthful alertness and premature senility and between overweight and youthful slimness.

Loses 30 Pounds in 46 Days With an Iodine Food

Helen G. wanted to lose 30 stubborn pounds. She tried group sessions, home exercises, and diet pills, but she kept on gaining weight. She found group sessions to be impersonal and embarrassing, and exercises made her hungrier! Diet pills made her feel sleepy, dizzy, and nauseous. She was resigned to being "unpleasingly plump" until she heard that a bariatrician (a physician who specializes in weight problems) was giving a talk at a local health club. He said that he would explain how a simple mineral, found in everyday food, could take pounds off and keep them off. So she went to hear the talk. She learned that the key to successful weight loss was in regulation of the thyroid. If she stimulated her sluggish thyroid, her thyroxine could increase metabolism and create internal "combustion" of accumulated fats, calories, and carbohydrates. The unsightly rolls of fat would actually "wash off" in a short time. A simple program was outlined.

Helen G. followed this basic program:

1. *Foods Should Be Fresh.* All foods should be fresh. Processed foods are very high in calories and deficient in iodine.

2. *Eat Seafood as Often as Possible.* Select a variety of different seafoods, especially deep-water seafoods. Seafood is a prime source of thyroid-activating iodine. Eat seafood daily if possible.

3. *Garlic: The Vegetable That Keeps You Slim.* Every day, Helen G. ate garlic. She diced it and added it to raw salads. She chopped it and added it to stews and soups. She used garlic powder (available at all food stores) as a seasoning. *Thyroid-Healing Benefit:* Garlic is one of the best iodine-containing plant foods available. The iodine is taken up by the body, stored by the thyroid, and used to stimulate production of fat-melting thyroxine. This youth serum uses the iodine to help speed up metabolism of accumulated weight in the body. It works from *within* to break up large particles of fat and remove them from the system.

4. *Use Sea Salt Daily.* Sea salt further fortified Helen G.'s metabolism with much-needed iodine. The iodine helped her sluggish thyroid create more fat-melting thyroxine so that pounds and inches could actually wash right out of her body.

Becomes Youthfully Slim. Day after day, Helen G. saw herself losing the stubborn fat. She weighed herself daily. She measured herself daily. Yes, the weight was washing right out of her system. Within 46 days, she had lost 30 unwanted pounds. She still follows this easy four-step program. She is youthfully slim. Thanks to an iodine-nourished thyroid, her internal "combustive" powers are alert and vigorous. Fat, calories, and carbohydrates are metabolized and burned up so that she can remain youthfully slim and healthy.

HOW TO REVITALIZE YOUR THYROID
IN 30 MINUTES

Boost the energy-creating powers of your thyroid in 30 minutes by drinking this tangy elixir:

Energy Elixir. Into a glass of tomato (or vegetable) juice, stir 1/2 teaspoon of kelp. Add 1/4 teaspoon of garlic powder. Stir vigorously and then drink slowly. Within 30 minutes, the iodine in this *Energy Elixir* will be taken up by the thyroid and used for the creation of the thyroxine that controls the speed at which all body activities occur.

You will feel more energy, more ambition, warm fingers and toes, and a healthier pulse rate.

Plan to take this *Energy Elixir* at least once daily so that your thyroid can release enough youth serum to keep you feeling alert, active, and alive!

From "Fat and Lazy" to "Slim and Peppy"

Sophie A. was fat and seemed lazy because her extra pounds made every job more difficult. She managed to take care of her family, but every chore was a major task. Every night she fell asleep in a chair, unable to participate in family talks or entertainment. In the morning it took a huge effort to get out of bed. She felt her strength slipping through her fingers, little by little.

Sophie A. felt that if she could lose weight she would feel more energetic. But the pounds clung stubbornly to her body. She could not get them off. Her eyelids felt as heavy as her shoulders, and she walked around looking half-asleep. She was well on the way to invalidism. Everyone was worried about her.

Biologist Outlines Four-Way Program. A biologist friend of her husband recognized the symptoms of a sluggish thyroid. He outlined a special four-way program that would help heal and revitalize her thyroid and give her much-needed pep and energy along with a loss of weight.

Sophie A. needed four ingredients to help alert and activate her sluggish thyroid: iodine, protein, B-complex vitamins, and Vitamin C. To obtain these four thyroid-boosting ingredients, she made the following tasty meal every night:

A seafood dish, either broiled or baked, according to taste.

A citrus fruit salad with a dressing made of two tablespoons of wheat germ oil and a squeeze of lemon juice.

One or two slices of whole grain bread.

A beverage consisting of a citrus juice with one tablespoon of wheat germ oil.

Thyroid-Revitalizing Benefit. This tasty meal offers four thryoid-revitalizing benefits that work in harmony.

1. The protein in the fish is metabolized into the amino acid tyrosine, out of which the thyroid youth serum thyroxine is made.

2. The tyrosine is activated and energized by the Vitamin C in the fruit salad, which prepares it in a form that can be used by the thyroid.

3. The vitamin E in the wheat germ oil and the whole grain bread

is needed to boost the absorption of iodine (from the fish) by the thyroid.

4. The Vitamin C in the citrus juice is needed to activate the thyroxine and prevent it from evaporating through oxygen exposure.

Simple Meal Is Slimming and Energizing. For 14 days, Sophie A. followed this simple program. Her runaway appetite subsided and came under her control. Day after day, pound after pound slipped away. Her pep and vigor returned slowly. She continued eating the simple main meal described above, varying it by using different seafoods prepared different ways with different sauces made out of oil, herbs, and spices. She also used different citrus fruits to satisfy her taste. At the end of 14 days, she had shed 27 pounds. Her attitude was cheerful. She felt so energetic that she was thinking about taking a part-time job to give herself "something to do." Thanks to this thyroid-boosting program, she went from "fat and lazy" to "slim and peppy" in just 14 days.

THYROID REVITALIZATION: KEY TO RENEWED YOUTH

Nourish your thyroid with iodine, and you will revitalize this organ so that it can give you the look and feel of renewed youth.

When iodine is metabolized and used to produce thyroxine, it helps revitalize your entire body at the same time.

The iodine-carrying youth serum will help improve the health of the thinking centers of your brain. It will also improve the health of your nervous system by neutralizing toxic wastes and joining with phosphorus to boost emotional health.

The iodine-carrying youth serum boosts assimilation of other nerve-feeding minerals and transports them to enrich the blood. The youth serum will increase the oxidation and elimination of impurities, improve mental activity because of rejuvenated brain functioning, and help protect the nervous system from shock by boosting the activity of the thyroid gland.

Rejuvenates From Head to Toe. The iodine-carrying youth serum protects the health of the skeletal and brain systems. It influences bone, teeth, and cellular metabolism. It promotes a favorable alkalinization of the saliva, oxidation of excess fat from the brain tissues, and removal of decomposed wastes from the brain. It influences the rate of the pulse, oxygenation of the brain, and removal of carbon dioxide from the brain and other body organs. The iodine-rich thyroxine youth serum can rejuvenate the body from head to toe.

Experience the joy of total revitalization with a well-nourished thyroid. With healthy foods, you can become superenergetic and youthfully slim, thanks to this small but influential organ.

HIGH POINTS

1. Thyroxine is the youth serum that peps you up in body and mind. Feed it iodine, and it will give you super energy and youthful slimness.
2. Earl McC. developed super energy on a tasty iodine-boosting diet.
3. Helen G. lost 30 pounds in 46 days and developed youthful vitality on a basic iodine-increasing diet.
4. Revitalize your thyroid in 30 minutes with a tangy *Energy Elixir.*
5. Sophie A. went from "fat and lazy" to "slim and peppy" in 14 days on a four-step iodine-boosting plan. She shed 27 unwanted pounds in those 14 days.
6. Iodine revitalizes your thyroid and rejuvenates your body from head to toe!

Your 21-Day Timetable for Internal Rejuvenation and Youthful Health

20

You are as youthful and healthy as your vital organs! These built-in "body motors" are the prime sources of youth serums, which help keep you looking and feeling alert, active, and youthfully alive! When you heal and revitalize your vital organs, you recharge these "body motors" so that they can send forth dynamic energy and health.

To rebuild these organs, plan a 21-day program. Each day, make a special improvement in your lifestyle. Little by little, your feelings of internal rejuvenation will emerge. Gradually, as day after day of improvement takes place, you will radiate the joys of youthful health. By the end of your 21-day program, you will feel alert, healthy, and brimming with the joy of life.

HOW TO PREPARE YOUR 21-DAY HEALTH TIMETABLE

1. *Set Your Goals.* Pick a set of 21 days that are convenient to you. No need to make any interruptions in your work or home schedule. You can continue your daily routine. You need only know that from the first day to the twenty-first day you will be making your various health adjustments.

2. *Prepare a Simple Daily Calendar.* Use a large calendar for making your 21 days. Below each day on your calendar, write the

233

health improvement you will follow on that day. List all 21 improvements. Have this calendar with you at all times so that you can plan ahead and also look backward to see how you are following the timetable.

3. *Change Gradually . . . Stick to Improvement.* Each day, you change gradually with this new health plan. Once you make the change, stick to this improvement as part of your program for daily living. For example, on one day you may decide that you will be good to your pancreas by eliminating refined sugar from your diet. You will kick the sugar habit on that day . . . and every day thereafter. Once you have made a change, stick to it!

4. *Check Your Health Progress Daily.* Note how your health improves as you make these permanent changes each day. If you feel that you need more improvement, increase a specific change if possible. For example, if you still have irregularity, increase the amount of bulk taken each day.

5. *Once You Begin Your 21-Day Timetable, Continue to End.* For optimum organ revitalization, plan to follow your 21-day timetable from the beginning to the end. Try not to skip any days or your healing and revitalization may be upset. Your rewards for perseverance will be the joys of youthful health from head to toe, inside and outside.

Now, here is your 21-day timetable. Start today!

First Day

Prepare your organs for change with a simple detoxifying program. On this first day, go on a raw vegetable juice fast. Drink as many different raw vegetable juices as you like, in any combination, throughout the day. Take on other foods. You will cleanse your organs and prepare your body for the healing and revitalization program to follow.

Second Day

Eliminate refined sugar in all forms. No matter what you are eating or drinking, it should be free of sugar. Use moderate amounts of honey, maple syrup, blackstrap molasses, or rose hips powder (available at health stores) as a sugar substitute.

Third Day

Eliminate salt and pepper and all other harsh seasonings in all forms. These include mustard, ketchup, and chemical seasonings.

Replace them with sea salt and natural herbs and spices. Be sure to read the labels of packaged foods. If they list salt or other volatile flavorings, avoid them. Retrain your taste buds to enjoy natural seasonings.

Fourth Day

Plan to do some moderate and comfortable exercises. If time permits, do some simple at-home exercises such as sit-ups, stretching, or knee-bends. Also plan to get outdoors (weather permitting) to walk at least 30 to 45 minutes in the morning and about one hour in the evening. Every day should include this exercise or walking.

Fifth Day

Alert and activate your organs with comfortable contrast baths. Use comfortably warm and comfortably cold water as you revitalize your circulation and boost the release of youth serums.

Sixth Day

Give up smoking. By now, you should feel stronger so that if you have a smoking urge you can give it up. If you feel giving up smoking is too difficult, taper off gradually by smoking one less cigarette each day.

Seventh Day

Give up drinking liquor in all forms. Switch to tangy vegetable juices to which you add lemon or lime juice. Calm down the drinking urge by adding a few ice cubes and a tablespoon of lime juice to tomato juice. Sprinkle some spices such as paprika over the drink to give your taste buds the illusion of hard liquor.

Eighth Day

Begin each of your main meals with a raw vegetable salad. Make a dressing of apple cider vinegar, and honey, oil; a scoop of cottage cheese or yogurt, or any fruit juice.

Ninth Day

Enjoy a lusciously sweet dessert in the form of fresh fruit, which you can further sweeten with some honey, maple syrup, or sun-dried raisins.

Tenth Day

Enjoy some sunshine today . . . and every day when it is possible. The warm rays of the sun will stimulate the oil glands beneath the surface of your skin into secreting important youth serums that boost basic body health. At least 30 minutes of controlled exposure to sun daily is helpful. Keep your head covered, though. Do not burn yourself.

Eleventh Day

Eliminate caffeine in all forms; that is, in coffee, soft drinks, commercial tea, cocoa, and chocolate. Switch to coffee substitutes (available at health stores), Postum, herbal teas, and carob-containing sweets (available at health stores), but read the labels. If the product contains sugar, pass it up.

Twelfth Day

Devote this entire day to raw fruit juices. This fasting program will help cleanse your organs of accumulated wastes and create better internal harmony.

Thirteenth Day

Go on a meat-free diet to give your organs a brief respite from their digestive tasks. Eat fresh or cooked vegetables in any combination. Baked eggplant and brown rice, for example, make an excellent main meal.

Fourteenth Day

Eat fresh fruits and vegetables and fish for your main meal. If possible, eat different types of fish for your three main meals.

Fifteenth Day

Eliminate all hard fats, including animal fats in any form. Trim away all visible fats before cooking and before eating meats. Switch to free-flowing, polyunsaturated vegetable oils. You can use some butter and margarine, but emphasize oils for all cooking and eating purposes.

Sixteenth Day

Air-wash your lungs with deep breathing. Do this whenever you feel tired. Be sure that you breathe in a pollution-free environment. Always keep your organs well ventilated for better health.

Seventeenth Day

Switch to whole grain bread, cereal, baked goods, and grains of any sort. Read package labels. If a product contains additives, bleached flour, sugar, or chemicals in any form, pass it up. Health stores and most supermarkets carry additive-free and sugar-free whole grain products.

Eighteenth Day

Find a quiet place where you can treat your organs to a little relaxation. Your entire body will react with refreshing health and stamina. About 30 minutes of soothing stillness can give you day-long energy and vigor.

Nineteenth Day

Go to your favorite restaurant and order a healthy, wholesome meal, based on the above suggestions. You'll find that most restaurants can offer you healthy, wholesome foods. Plan to eat natural and wholesome foods in restaurants whenever you dine out.

Twentieth Day

Immerse yourself in a tub of comfortably warm water at night. Add fragrances in the form of herbs and scents, which are available at all supermarkets, pharmacies, and health stores. Luxuriate and indulge yourself for 30 minutes.

Twenty-first Day

Each night, plan to enjoy at least eight hours of refreshing sleep. Do not skimp or deny yourself sleep, or you will pay the toll in organ decline and loss of health.

LOOK YOUNGER, FEEL REJUVENATED, AND
ENJOY LIFE

At the end of your 21-day timetable, you will look younger, feel rejuvenated and be filled with the desire to enjoy the best that life has to offer. These are only some of your rewards for having healed and revitalized your organs. As the days pass, you will discover that life can be a joy, thanks to your revitalized health.

Your body organs are like intricately patterned printed circuits within your human machine. Each organ is a link in a chain. The malfunctioning or weakening of just one organ can bring down the entire chain and cause the collapse of the entire human machine.

That is why your health program is aimed at healing and revitalizing your body organs. They are the very foundations of your health. When they all work in harmony, the body machine throbs with vitality and youthful health.

Heal and revitalize your body organs, and you will create the foundation for radiant rejuvenation, better health, and longer life.

Organ-Healer Locator Index